THE BRAIN IN HOMINID
EVOLUTION

PHILLIP V. TOBIAS

The brain in hominid evolution

 COLUMBIA UNIVERSITY PRESS
NEW YORK & LONDON

1971

Phillip V. Tobias is Professor of Anatomy at the University of the Witwatersrand, Johannesburg.

This book is based on the author's James Arthur Lecture, delivered at the American Museum of Natural History, New York City, April 30, 1969; it was the thirty-eighth in this series of lectures.

Copyright © 1971 Columbia University Press
International Standard Book Number: 0-231-03518-7
Library of Congress Catalog Card Number: 78-158458
Printed in the United States of America

JAMES ARTHUR LECTURES ON THE EVOLUTION OF THE HUMAN BRAIN

v

* Published versions of these lectures can be obtained from The American Museum of Natural History, Central Park West at 79th St., New York, N. Y. 10024.

† Published for The American Museum of Natural History by Columbia University Press.

FOREWORD

It can scarcely be denied that the development of the brain is a central, even a determining, aspect of human evolution. For, as we learn more about this process, it becomes increasingly evident that the changes leading to *Homo sapiens* are intimately linked in a kind of feedback situation with the brain. Even if we knew nothing else about it, its threefold increase in size during hominid evolution would merit, if not demand, a special interest. And yet this is one of the least known of the adaptive changes that have occurred in human evolution.

One obvious reason, but not the only one, for this is that the brain does not fossilize and thereby provides us, as do the bony and dental structures, with an anatomical record that would enable us to trace in some detail its development. All that we do have in the way of fossil evidence is the inner surface molding and the capacity of the braincase. And the latter can be inferred by indirect methods only for the many cases where the fossil specimen is fragmentary.

But because our evidence is so limited, what we do have, or can reasonably be inferred, takes on an enhanced importance, and it is essential that it be properly and meticulously assembled and appraised. For much can be learned and certain deductions of great importance may be drawn from such data. This necessary task has been admirably carried out by Professor Tobias in his James Arthur Lecture, now expanded in the following book. His broad experience with hominid fossil material has richly equipped him for this task. We are all deeply indebted to him for this valuable survey, long overdue, which I predict will be a standard reference for a long time.

Harry L. Shapiro

PREFACE

This little volume grew out of the thirty-eighth James Arthur Lecture on the Evolution of the Human Brain, which I delivered at the American Museum of Natural History, New York City, on 30 April 1969. There are many ways to approach brain evolution, including the electrophysiological, comparative, ontogenetic, and neurochemical. My choice of a direction, conditioned by my own background as an anatomist and palaeoanthropologist, fell on "Some Aspects of the *Fossil Evidence* on the Evolution of the Hominid Brain." This choice confined me to two phases: the gross external morphology of the brain (as reflected by the modeling of, and markings on, the interior of the braincase and by endocranial casts, natural and artificial) and the tangible evidence of what hominids could do with their brains, in the form of artefacts and other cultural objects.

The study of gross external morphology was further circumscribed: it was confined to the measurable. Of all the quantifiable aspects of the brain, its overall size is perhaps the parameter that can be determined most readily and most objectively. Moreover, brain size is highly relevant for such a study as it shows evidence of dramatic change during hominid evolution. Of course, in fossil studies we are unable to determine brain size as such; we are able to measure only the size of the braincase, the endocranial capacity (often loosely called the cranial capacity). Although much tissue and fluid intervene between the brain and the bony walls of the cranial vault, there is obviously a relationship between the size and shape of the two, variable though it may be. Following normal development, big brains lie in big cranial vaults and small brains in small vaults.

In selecting size as my yardstick of change in gross encephalic morphology, I was, of course, aware of the work of numerous investigators who have addressed themselves to other external morphological features, (e.g. Le Gros Clark, Cooper, and Zuckerman 1936; Edinger 1948; Connolly 1950; Simon 1965; Bauchot and Stephan 1967). Such features have included the lobes and areas of the cerebrum, the positions of certain key fissures, the detailed pattern of convolutions and sulci—and what has been rather inelegantly described by some as "the degree of sulcification" or "the degree of fissuration." I was aware, too, of the considerable subjective element that has often entered into such studies, especially when applied to inter-racial comparisons; of the fact that it is most difficult, and for some characters virtually impossible, to express such observations in precise metrical form; and of the comment by the distinguished neuroanatomist, Dr. Gerhardt von Bonin, after a lifetime of studies on brains and endocasts: "It should at last be admitted that most of what has been said and written on the sulci of the brain as they have been seen on endocasts is worth very little" (von Bonin 1963, p. 50), a view that is shared by not a few of those mentioned above. These are among the reasons why I have chosen to confine this study to brain size and endocranial capacity.

It started, as I have said, as a single lecture and, as such, possesses a single unifying theme. Briefly stated, it is this: nothing is more striking and more sustained in the whole of human evolution than the twofold trend towards increase in brain size on the one hand, and, on the other, towards cultural activities, cultural mastery, and, indeed, utter dependence on culture for survival. These two sets of changes are indissolubly linked. The chain between them may be set forth simply as follows: increase in brain size $\rightleftharpoons$ gain in intricacy of neuronal organization $\rightleftharpoons$ rise in complexity of nervous function $\rightleftharpoons$ ever more diversified and complicated behavior responses $\rightleftharpoons$ progressively amplified and enhanced cultural manifestations.

This essay explores the first and last steps of this causal chain—the steps that are directly manifest in the fossil record. It pleads that these two items are valid fields of study, each in its own right, irrespective of the tangled skein that may connect them. With Stephan (1969), this essay accepts that "The functional capacity of a system depends upon its size and *structural differentiation*" (italics mine); that, in addition, "The two variables of struc-ture—size and differentiation—in general do not vary independently," but that ". . . the *differentiation* can vary in many ways (e.g. in construction, arrangements and connection of the cells, units, layers, etc.), whereas for variations in *size* there are only two possibilities: enlargement or reduction" (Stephan 1969, p. 34). This work fully recognizes the importance of the intervening areas of knowledge. In fact, it very gingerly peers into the murky fastnesses of the fossil neuron, the glia-neuron ratio and relationship, the feedback chains, and other components of the middle links that will one day establish the logic and the causality uniting the termini. Into this no-man's land, at present, only the intrepid few are venturing. It is in these

x

intervening areas that the next major chapter in the history of the brain in hominid evolution waits to be written.

Meantime, this little book attempts to marshal and evaluate the crucial evidence at the two ends of the chain: for accurate observation and cautious interpretation of these relatively simple and modest first criteria are the foundations upon which any later, profounder study must be predicated.

Johannesburg, December 1970   *P. V. Tobias*

ACKNOWLEDGMENTS

This work was made possible through the generosity of Professor R. A. Dart, Dr. and Mrs. L. S. B. Leakey, Dr. G. H. R. von Koenigswald, Dr. D. Hooijer, and Dr. J. T. Wiebes.

I express my thanks to Miss C. J. Orkin, Mrs. J. Asch, Mrs. E. Judd, and Mrs. E. Hibbett, for their painstaking preparation of the manuscript; to Mr. A. R. Hughes, Mr. B. Hume, and Mr. M. Hockman, for preparation of the illustrations; and to Mr. R. J. Clarke, Mr. C. Block, and Miss S. Etoe for other assistance.

The original researches reported in this volume were subvented by the Research Committee of the University of the Witwatersrand, the Council for Scientific and Industrial Research of South Africa, the Wenner-Gren Foundation for Anthropological Research, the National Science Foundation, and the Boise Fund.

I am indebted to Dr. Harry L. Shapiro for kindly writing the Foreword, to the American Museum of Natural History for according me the honor of inviting me to deliver the thirty-eighth James Arthur Lecture; and especially to Dr. Shapiro and Dr. Lester R. Aronson for their kindness and assistance.

Finally, I sincerely appreciate the patient and friendly cooperation of those many people at the Columbia University Press—and particularly the editor, Mrs. Barbara-Jo Kawash—who have collaborated superbly in producing this little book. It has been a pleasure to work with them.

CONTENTS

THE BRAIN IN HOMINID
EVOLUTION

ONE

OF BRAINS, MEN, AND FOSSILS

Probably no branch of biology is more charged with immoderate, emotive, and misleading statements than that which deals with man himself. It is likely, too, that few branches of human biology are more bedeviled with half truths, selective omissions, and the forthright proclamation of unproved propositions than that which deals with brain size and, especially, the relationship between brain size and function.

It is not surprising, therefore, that when these two fields converge in the physical anthropology of the brain some interesting departures from scientific methodology and logic occur. Often, indeed, it seems that the techniques of the scientist give way, in greater or lesser measure, to those of the publicist and the propagandist.

These difficulties characterize the study of brains among living peoples, where material is abundant and where both brains and behavior can be studied directly. When we deal with fossil man the problems are multiplied a hundredfold, for in the main, evidence is scanty and embraces only the size and shape of endocranial casts, or the capacity of the braincase, supplemented by the fossilized signs of behavior, such as material culture.

Small wonder, therefore, that the history of such studies shows some dramatic swings of the pendulum: from an optimistic extreme at which it has been claimed that functional areas can be identified on endocasts with relative ease, to a gloomy opposite pole at which it has been averred that endocasts can teach us practically nothing at all.

In this volume I shall try to dissect out the facts about brain size, cranial capacity, and the fossil evidence of behavior. Some of the facts will be culled from the literature; others will be based upon original studies I have been privileged to make upon most of the original fossil hominid crania from Africa, Asia, and Europe.

At the outset, lest I give the impression of sailing under false colors, let me make clear that I am no neurologist, but rather a simple anatomist, with some anthropological and genetical experience, who is trying to apply himself to the study of ancient as well as modern anatomies. My thinking lacks the

1

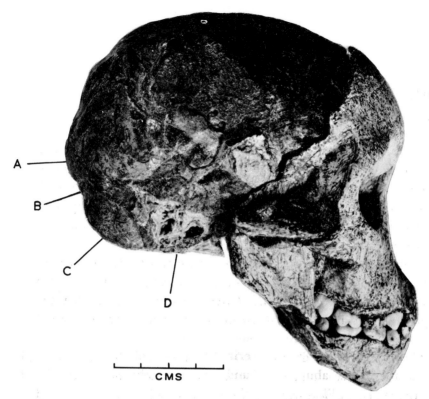

FIGURE 1: Right lateral view of the Taung skull, type specimen of *Austra-lopithecus africanus*. The endocast is beautifully preserved and shows much detail of convolutional and vascular impressions. (A) impression of occipital pole of cerebrum; (B) impression of right lateral sinus, curving over the cerebellum; (C) impression of cerebellar hemisphere; (D) portion of petrous temporal bone preserved between impressions of cerebellum and temporal lobe of cerebrum.

elegant concepts of modern neurology, and I blanch before the ever more refined techniques being focussed on the central nervous system. Brains are being studied by electron microscopy, biochemical analyses, autoradiography, ultraviolet absorption spectromicrophotometry, cybernetic models, tissue culture, and a host of other methods.

It seems incomprehensible, in the light of such developments, that anything at all remains to be said about so gross and crude a measure as the overall size of the brain. But it is an amazing yet inescapable fact that a great deal remains to be said, for much that has already been asserted about the brain size of both fossil man and the living races does not stand up to the cold light of scientific scrutiny.

The cranial capacity as a measure of brain size

When we deal with fossils and recent dried skulls we are not able to determine the size of the brain but only that of the braincase, or calvaria.

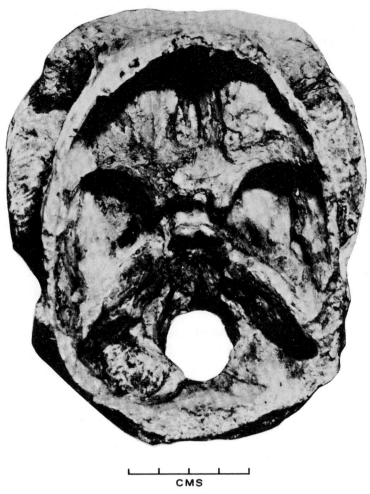

CMS

FIGURE 2: Interior of the base of the cranium of *Australopithecus africanus* from Sterkfontein (Sts 5). It is possible to make an artificial endocast of plaster of Paris or other medium, where the cranium has not become filled with matrix.

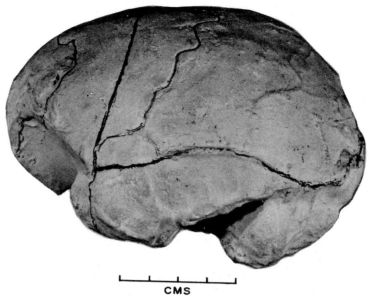

CMS

FIGURE 3: Artificial plaster endocast of *Australopithecus boisei* (Olduvai hominid 5). The portion of the endocast between the two wavy lines in front has been restored, as the bony wall of the vault was missing in this region. The outline of the parietal bone has been drawn on the endocast.

We may have a natural endocranial cast formed as a result of the braincase becoming filled with sand or other matrix, which in turn becomes consolidated by some such impregnating medium as lime (Figure 1). This is likely to occur wherever fossils are preserved in dolomitic limestone cave deposits, and it is true of several of the South African deposits, such as Taung, Sterkfontein, and Swartkrans, containing remains of the early hominid, the ape-man *Australopithecus*.

In other situations the braincase may have failed to fill with matrix after death, and we are presented with an empty cranium (Figure 2). Under these circumstances, with no supporting material inside the braincase, the cranium is frequently found broken or crushed. From an intact braincase, or from a reconstruction of one, it is possible to make an artificial endocast with plaster of Paris or some other medium such as gelatin (Zuckerman 1928) or latex (Radinsky 1968). This has been done, for instance, with the early hominid crania we have assigned to *Australopithecus boisei* (Tobias

1967a) and *Homo habilis* (Leakey, Tobias, and Napier 1964) from Olduvai (Figure 3).

Both a natural and an artificial endocast take faithful impressions of all markings on the interior of the braincase. For example, the meningeal arteries and the cranial venous sinuses leave clear imprints on the inside of the vault-bones of the cranium (Figure 4). So do the major subdivisions of the brain, such as the cerebrum, the cerebellum, and to a certain extent the brainstem (Figure 5).

Finer subdivisions of the brain may leave their mark as well; for example, the convolutions of the cerebral cortex and the sulci separating them are responsible for the well-known *impressiones gyrorum* on the inner surface of the vault-bones. All these features are, in turn, reflected sensitively on an endocast, whether natural or artificial. Sometimes the filling material in a natural endocast extends into one or more of the foramina in the base

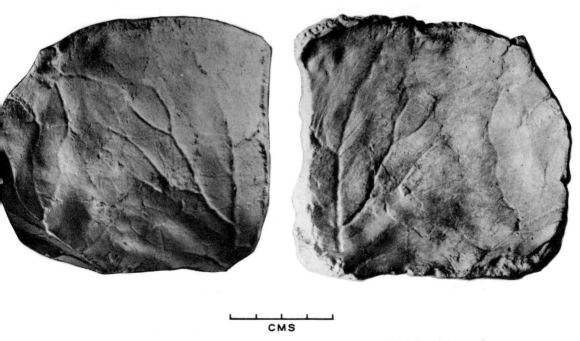

CMS

FIGURE 4: The parietal bone of Ternifine, Morocco (*right*) with a plaster impression of its endocranial surface (*left*). Note the clearly marked impressions left by the branches of the middle meningeal artery. The group of Middle Pleistocene hominid remains from Ternifine has been classified as *Homo erectus*.

5 🖋

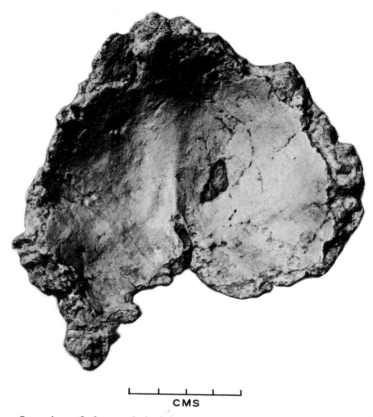

CMS

FIGURE 5: Interior of the occipital bone of Vértèsszöllös, Hungary, showing clear impressions for both the cerebral and the cerebellar hemispheres.

of the calvaria and takes a cast of the little bony canal to which the foramen gives access. Since most of the foramina transmit cranial nerves or their branches, we may even have thus a cast representing one or two of the bigger cranial nerves coming off the brainstem (Figure 6).

In addition, the sutures or linear joints between 2 adjacent vault-bones —such as the coronal suture between the frontal and parietal bones, the sagittal suture between the left and the right parietal bones and the lamb-doid suture between the parietal bones and the occipital—generally leave a clear imprint on the endocast, if by the time of the individual's death these sutures had not begun to fuse (Figure 7).

Once formed and consolidated, an endocranial cast is a tough and durable structure. Often it may outlast damage to, or loss of, the surrounding bone, as is true of the Taung child's endocast and the newest hominid endocast from Swartkrans.

Thus, an endocast—though simply a concretion of matrix—is full of character. And, too, it may reflect antemortem injury to a cranium, such as a depressed fracture (Figure 8).

Both natural and artificial endocasts provide us with a ready means of determining the capacity of a fossil cranium. A third method may be employed when a cranium is empty and is reasonably intact: the cranium may be filled with a relatively slightly compressible medium such as millet seed. The volume of seed required to fill the brainpan may then be determined.

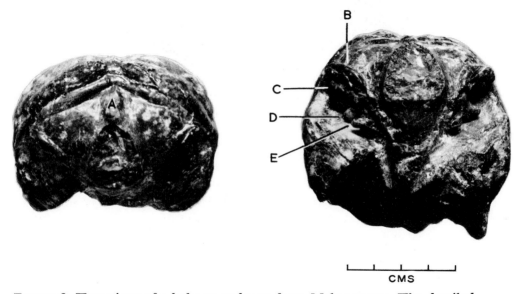

FIGURE 6: Two views of a baboon endocast from Makapansgat. The detailed anatomy of this part of the brain had been vividly etched on the endocranium, making possible the formation of this superb natural endocast. (A) impression of vermis of cerebellum; (B) impression of sigmoid sinus coursing over the surface of the cerebellar hemisphere; (C) impression of antero-lateral pole of cerebellar hemisphere; (D) impression of the large subarcuate fossa which characterizes the posterior surface of the petrous temporal of cercopithecoids; (E) impression of the internal acoustic meatus—in effect, this stump represents the seventh (facial) and eighth (vestibulo-cochlear) nerves.

7 🖋

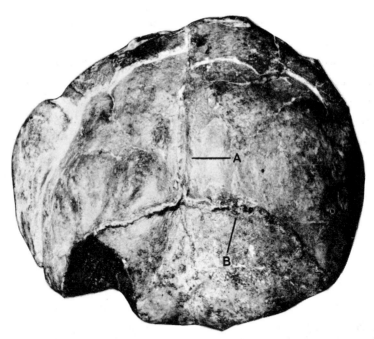

FIGURE 7: Partial endocast of *Australopithecus africanus* from Sterkfontein, to show the clear markings of the sagittal suture (A) and of the lambdoid suture (B).

As standardized, for example, by Breitinger (1936), this method has been widely used in studies on long series of modern skulls.

All three methods—the determination of the volume of a natural and of an artificial endocast, and the determination of the capacity of the braincase —provide one with an assessment of the volume of the space within the cranium. They do *not* provide us with the volume of the brain as such. For it must be remembered that the cranial cavity accommodates a great deal more than simply brain. Thus, when we say that a skull has an endocranial capacity of 1400 c.c., this includes the roots and intracranial trunks of no fewer than 24 cranial nerves, the thick outer brain covering, or dura mater, the 2 thinner coverings, or leptomeninges, namely the arachnoid and pia mater, the subarachnoid space and its enlargements, the cisterns, containing cerebrospinal fluid, numerous blood vessels including larger meningeal and cerebral arteries and veins, and the enlarged venous channels called cranial venous sinuses, blood, and cerebrospinal fluid.

Thus, only a proportion of the cranial capacity is made up of brain tissue: estimates of this proportion vary. On the one hand we have Wingate Todd's (1923, p. 265) statement, "Of course it is impossible to ascertain how fully the brain ever occupies the total possible space at its disposal." On the other hand figures are cited ranging from 10 per cent (Brandes 1927) to as high as 33⅓ per cent (cited by Mettler in his 1955 *James Arthur Lecture*).

Cranial capacity is therefore only an approximation to the size of the brain itself. It might be deemed that we could simply apply a correction factor to the determined capacity in order to ascertain the brain size. Unfortunately, the wide discrepancy between the 2 extreme figures cited—10 per cent and 33⅓ per cent—would vitiate such a correction. Furthermore, the ratio is not a constant figure within the adult lifetime of any one individual, for the brain shrinks with age, in certain illnesses, and under some other

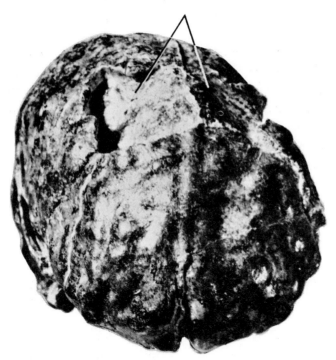

FIGURE 8: Antero-superior view of a natural endocast of a presumed *Australopithecus africanus* from Sterkfontein. The pointers indicate a pair of localized impressions where the surface of the endocast drops below the surrounding intact surface, consequent upon a doubly indented depressed fracture of the cranium. All trace of bone has since disappeared, leaving only the indented surface of the endocast.

TABLE 1: *Age changes in the ratio of brain volume to cranial capacity in modern man* [a]	Age	Volume of brain (in c.c.)	Cranial capacity (in c.c.)	Percentage
	Newborn	330	350	94.3
	3 months	500	600	83.3
	6 months	575	775	74.2
	9 months	675	925	73.0
	1 year	750	1000	75.0
	2 years	900	1100	81.8
	3 years	960	1225	78.4
	4 years	1000	1300	76.9
	6 years	1060	1350	78.5
	9 years	1100	1400	78.6
	12 years	1150	1450	79.3
	20 years	1200	1500	80.0

[a] Calculated by ourselves from the data in *Tabulae Biologicae*, 1941.

conditions, and swells under yet other circumstances, though the braincase itself has not been shown to diminish in capacity (Anderson 1910; Stillman 1911; Zuckerman 1928; Appel and Appel 1942; Tobias 1970). Hence, as the quality and duration of life change, the non-neural endocranial capacity increases, and one's head becomes filled more and more with fluid and meninges (Anderson 1910; Stillman 1911; Todd 1923; Greenfield and Carmichael 1925; Zuckerman 1928).

We know a little of the percentage of the cavity occupied by non-neural contents at different ages (Donaldson 1895, Bolk 1904, Rudolph 1914, cited by Zuckerman 1928). What correction should we apply, for example, to the cranial capacity of the Taung child who had just reached the stage of erupting his first permanent molar tooth, that is, an age of perhaps five or six years? And what correction to Sterkfontein 5 who was old enough for the sutures of her cranium largely to have closed? How much for the capacity of Olduvai hominid 5 (*A. boisei*, formerly called *Zinjanthropus*), who died as an adolescent with incompletely erupted wisdom teeth (third molars)? We can arrive at only approximate answers to these questions on the age variations in the ratio of brain size to cranial capacity.

Some lead is given by a table published in *Tabulae Biologicae*, 1941. For a series of ages from birth to twenty years, the table cites the volume of the brain, the cranial capacity, and the weight of the brain. The figures in our Table 1 are extracted from this source. The capacity of the cranium in the newborn infant is cited as 1.01 to 1.06 times as great as the volume of the brain, but at the age of one year as 1.3 times as great (Blinkov and Glezer 1968). Siwe (1931), however, reports that the change is less marked. The figures cited in Table 1 show that, by twenty years of age, no more than 80 per cent of the endocranial cavity is occupied by brain. These figures have, of course, been determined on modern man. Even if we could accept them as adequate and consistent results for modern *Homo sapiens,* we could not lightly assume that the same percentages would apply to earlier hominids at the same ages. The rate of growth of brain may have been different—and we shall return to this theme when we discuss the work of Krantz (1961) in Chapter 11. Moreover, the rate of growth of the non-neural contents of the cranial cavity, as well as the rate of growth of the braincase itself, may have differed. With all these possible variables entering into the picture, we certainly would be unwise to take for granted that the percentage differences reflected in the figures taken from *Tabulae Biologicae* would have applied, age for age, to *Australopithecus* or any other early hominid.

Our ignorance goes still deeper. Brandes showed that modern man's brain contains as much as 50 gms. of cerebrospinal fluid before draining, while the dura mater weighs on the average 50 to 60 gms. (Brandes 1927) and has a volume of about 50 to 60 c.c. (Rudolph 1914). We shall never know if similar values applied to *Australopithecus* and other extinct hominids; and so we shall never be able to determine the brain size of fossil man with precision.

We shall have to rest content with the cranial capacity, recognizing that this is only an approximation of the brain size. Through most of this book I shall be dealing with this inexact parameter, cranial capacity, but I hope to show that the changes that have occurred in cranial capacity have been of such a magnitude as to point to an undoubted dramatic increase in true brain size during hominid evolution.

TWO

 # THE CRANIAL CAPACITY OF THE AUSTRALOPITHECINES

Of all the fossil crania assigned to the South and East African fossil ape-man genus, *Australopithecus* sensu lato, only 8 specimens are sufficiently complete and undistorted to permit a reasonable assessment of their endocranial capacity. These 8 specimens exclude those Olduvai crania that have been assigned as type and paratypes of the larger-brained group, which Leakey, Tobias, and Napier (1964) have called *Homo habilis*.

Seven of these 8 australopithecine specimens are from South Africa—4 from Sterkfontein, 1 from Taung, 1 from Makapansgat, and 1 from Swartkrans—whilst the eighth specimen is from Olduvai. Those from Sterkfontein, Taung, and Makapansgat are generally regarded as belonging to the gracile species, *A. africanus* (Robinson 1956), though Tobias (1967a, 1968a) has drawn attention to certain features of the Makapansgat specimens that suggest a degree of intermediacy between the gracile and robust forms. The specimen from Swartkrans is of a robust australopithecine, *A. robustus* (sometimes regarded as a separate genus, *Paranthropus*); whilst that from Olduvai is the type specimen of the hyper-robust species, *A. boisei* (Tobias 1967a). Thus, we have 6 estimates of cranial capacity for *A. africanus*, and 1 each for *A. robustus* and *A. boisei*. Let us consider the individual data.

The gracile australopithecines

THE TAUNG CHILD SKULL. This beautifully preserved skull is the type specimen of *A. africanus* (Dart 1925). It includes a well-preserved natural endocranial cast (Figure 1). The endocast comprises the impression of virtually all of the right cerebral hemisphere, though the frontal pole and adjacent rostral region are broken off from the main body of the endocast and remain embedded against the frontal bone and the anterior cranial fossa. Posteriorly, the endocast stops short of the midline, the plane of cleavage diverging from the median sagittal plane and approaching close to the impression of the right cerebellar hemisphere. Thus, a sufficient amount of the endocast is preserved to permit a fair reconstruction to be made of the hemicast and of the entire cast.

In his original paper, it is of interest to note that Professor Dart gave no estimate of the cranial capacity; he gave an estimate of the length of the cranial cavity ("could not have been less than 114 mm.") and made certain comparisons with the cranial cavity of a chimpanzee skull and with a large endocast of a gorilla. From these statements, Sir Arthur Keith made a rough estimate of the approximate "brain volume" (i.e., endocranial capacity), namely, "less than 450 c.c." (Keith 1925, p. 234).

In his 1926 paper in *Natural History*, Dart stated that the endocranial volume was 520 c.c. The reconstruction of the hemi-endocast on which this computation was based is still present in the Anatomy Department of the

Witwatersrand University, labeled 260 c.c. (for the half-volume). A cast of this reconstructed endocast was presented by Dart to University College, London, where Zuckerman (1928) determined the volume of the total endocast to be 500 c.c. Dart's (1929) paper cited no figure for the capacity.

Keith stated that he had made "an exact model of half the brain" in plasticine. It measured 225 c.c., giving 450 c.c. for the whole as "a minimum size." Nevertheless, he was prepared to take 500 c.c. as "an impartial estimate," and, in addition, he used the figure of 500 c.c. in computing the "adult size" for Taung (Keith 1931, pp. 61–65).

Two decades after the first publication Schepers (1946) attempted further reconstructions and reported that they "gave results which varied but little from this figure (500 c.c.)," which he stated, not quite precisely, was that earlier claimed for it by Dart. As mentioned above, Dart's original claim was 520 c.c. In fact, Schepers used the figure of 500 c.c. in his text (p. 238) and of 520 c.c. in his Table 1 (p. 242).

Le Gros Clark in 1947 stated that "Zuckerman's estimate of 500 c.c. is sufficiently close [to Dart's original estimate] to be taken as confirmatory" (Le Gros Clark 1947, p. 313). Still later, Le Gros Clark (1964, p. 133) described the capacity as "rather more than 500 c.c."

On the basis of these estimates by Dart, Zuckerman, Schepers, and Le Gros Clark, I have cited 500 to 520 c.c. for the volume in my tables of estimates of australopithecine cranial capacities (Tobias 1963, 1967a).

Working in our Anatomy Department, Dr. R. L. Holloway, Jr. has recently reopened the question of the cranial capacity of the Taung child, and his new provisional reconstruction gives a smaller value.* With estimates ranging on either side of 500 c.c., it would seem to be safest, for the time being, to accept 500 c.c. as an approximation of the cranial capacity of the Taung child.

The problem now arises of what cranial capacity the Taung individual would have attained had he lived to adulthood. Dart was keenly aware of

---

* Since the James Arthur Lecture was delivered, Holloway (1970b) has published his new estimate for the endocranial capacity of the Taung child. Based on new reconstructions made by him in the Anatomy Department in 1969, he has arrived at a figure of 405 c.c., the mean of the capacities of his 2 most accurate reconstructions. This figure is well below the figure of 500 to 520 c.c. accepted by most workers up to the present but is closer to Sir Arthur Keith's original rough estimate of "less than 450 c.c." When Holloway's estimate of 405 c.c. is corrected for the juvenile age of the Taung child, he obtains an adult estimate of 440 c.c., exactly 100 c.c. less than the latest adult estimate based on the old reconstruction.

this problem as long ago as 1925. In his now classic announcement of the Taung discovery, he stated:

Few data are available concerning the expansion of brain matter which takes place in the living anthropoid brain between the time of eruption of the first permanent molars and the time of their becoming adult. So far as man is concerned, Owen (*Anatomy of Vertebrates* vol. iii) tells us that "The brain has advanced to near its term of size at about ten years, but it does not usually obtain its full development till between twenty and thirty years of age." R. Boyd (1860) discovered an increase in weight of nearly 250 grams in the brains of male human beings after they had reached the age of seven years. [Dart 1925, p. 197]

However, in this first paper, as mentioned before, Dart ventured no estimate of the capacity, either of the child or of the adult. Keith, in his comment in *Nature* a week later, did make an estimate. He stated that in the fourth year a human child has reached 81 per cent of the total size of its brain, whilst, "at the same period," a young gorilla has attained 85 per cent of its full brain size and a chimpanzee 87 per cent. No statement was made about the sample size nor the origin of the materials upon which these statements were based. From these figures Keith chose the value of 85 per cent to apply to the *Australopithecus* endocast. Based on his estimate of "less than 450 c.c.," he computed that the adult brain "will not exceed 520 c.c." (Keith 1925).

In his *Natural History* paper, Dart (1926) gave his estimate of 520 c.c. for the child and added 20 per cent, which he described as "a reasonable amount to allow for subsequent expansion." This gave him an adult estimate of 625 c.c.

Zuckerman (1928) based his estimates on chimpanzee data and pointed out that, by analogy with the chimpanzee, the subsequent growth would have varied with the sex. The average expansion, he stated, after the eruption of the first molar is 8.1 per cent in the chimpanzee, regardless of sex. In the male the average expansion was given as 11.3 per cent, and in the female as 3 per cent. The final capacities estimated by Zuckerman for a Taung adult were therefore as follows:

regardless of sex	540 c.c.
if male	566 c.c.
if female	515 c.c.

These figures, as will be seen, are remarkably similar to those obtained by my latest estimates based on newer comparative material.

Keith's later detailed study led him to an upward revision of his earlier estimate: namely to 600 c.c. This figure was an increase of 20 per cent and was based on Keith's own study of the growth of cranial capacity in gorillas (Keith 1931, p. 65).

The figure of 600 c.c. was accepted too by Le Gros Clark (1964), although he had earlier (1947) used Zuckerman's (1928) data on chimpanzees to estimate an adult size of about 570 c.c. (or rather more, if Dart's estimate of 520 c.c. for the child were accepted as the basis).

In 1958 Ashton and Spence published a new important contribution on the cranial capacity at various ages in several living species of the Hominoidea. They found that by the time the first molar has erupted endocranial capacity has reached 94 per cent of adult size in man and chimpanzee, 91 to 92 per cent in orangutan, and 90 per cent in gorilla. Thus, for this group of hominoids the mean values fluctuate narrowly between 90 and 94 per cent. The unweighted mean percentage for the 4 kinds of living hominoids is 92.5.

On the basis of this intergroup mean of 92.5 per cent I recomputed the "adult value" for Taung as 562 c.c. (Tobias 1965a). For this estimation I employed the juvenile value of 520 c.c. based on Dart (1926) and Schepers (1946, Table 1). I now feel that it would be safer to accept the juvenile value of no more than 500 c.c., as found by Zuckerman (1928) and Schepers (1946, p. 238, in text). On the basis of this figure of 500 c.c. and the correction factor of 92.5 per cent derived from Ashton and Spence (1958), one arrives at the adult value for Taung of 540 c.c.* This happens to be exactly the same figure that Zuckerman had arrived at on the basis of his chimpanzee data in 1928, when sex differences were not taken into account.

The figure of 540 c.c. is therefore tentatively accepted by me as the nearest approach we can make with present information, and with the reconstructions of Dart and Schepers, to the adult endocranial capacity of the Taung creature. The figure should now replace such previous estimates in the literature as 562, 570, and 625 c.c. It should be stressed that I have made no new reconstruction of the endocast but have based my computations on Dart's original reconstruction—which was acceptable to Zuckerman, Schepers, and Le Gros Clark. Needless to say, other reconstructions are possible, which would yield varying estimates of the child's total cranial capacity and, hence, of the adult value. Holloway's new reconstruction is an example.

---

* Holloway (1970b) used the figure of 92.0 per cent to compute an adult estimate of 440 c.c. from the capacity of his new reconstruction (405 c.c.).

THE STERKFONTEIN CRANIA. Four crania or endocasts from Sterkfontein have permitted reasonable determinations or estimates of endocranial capacity to be made. The most complete and perfectly preserved cranium was that of Sterkfontein skull Sts 5 (Figure 2). Broom and Robinson (1950) estimated its capacity as 482 c.c., and Schepers (1950) and Robinson (1954) accepted the figure of 480.* The latter figure was used by me in several tabulations (1963, 1967a, 1968b).†

"Skull 8" from Sterkfontein comprises much of the top of the braincase (Sts 58) and a well-preserved base (Sts 19). From these 2 parts, Broom and Robinson (1948) reconstructed the whole endocast "with considerable confidence," yielding a value of about 530 c.c. This figure I employed in my tabulations (Tobias 1963, 1967a, 1968b). Schepers, however, cited values for this specimen of 550 to 570 c.c. in his Table 1 (1950); he did not explain how his reconstruction came to be so much larger in volume than that of Broom and Robinson. If the value of 530 c.c. is correct, this would give Sterkfontein 8 the biggest capacity of the Sterkfontein australopithecines whose capacities have so far been determined or estimated, and of all the gracile australopithecines, save that the Taung "adult value" is 540 c.c.‡

The capacity of the very complete Sterkfontein 1 endocast (the type specimen of what was earlier called *Plesianthropus*), now catalogued as Sts 60, was estimated by Schepers (1946) as 435 c.c. and by Broom and Robinson (1948) as about 450 c.c. Le Gros Clark (1947, 1964) considered Schepers' estimate of 435 c.c. "reasonable" and "fairly reliable," and I have employed this figure in my own tables.§

* Earlier, Broom and Robinson (1948) had spoken of the capacity of "the beautiful female skull" (presumably the same Sts 5 cranium) as being about 415 c.c. Their upgrading of this figure appeared in the 1950 monograph.

† Holloway (1970b) has recently confirmed this volume, obtaining an estimate of 485 c.c. for the capacity of the artificial endocast.

‡ Holloway (1970b) has recently published a new estimate of 436 c.c., based on the partial endocast of Sts 19, the base of this cranium. Broom and Robinson (1948) and Schepers (1950) used both the base (Sts 19) and the calotte (Sts 58) to reconstruct an entire endocast for which they obtained values of about 530 c.c. and 550 to 570 c.c., respectively. However, as Holloway (personal communication) points out, in neither instance were the methods of reconstruction and of volume determination well described by these earlier workers. Holloway (1970b and personal communication) did not attempt a reconstruction based on both parts of this cranium (Sts 19 and Sts 58) but made separate estimates based, respectively, on each of the 2 parts. He considers his estimates based on the calotte (Sts 58) to be most tentative and insecure, whereas he is more confident about the value estimated from the endocast of the basis cranii (Sts 19), that is, 436 c.c. It is this last figure alone that is quoted in his paper (Holloway 1970b).

§ Holloway has recently confirmed this figure, with an estimate of 428 c.c.

🌿 16

The fourth Sterkfontein cranium to yield an estimate of cranial capacity is that designated Sterkfontein 7 in the 1950 monograph by Broom and Robinson. It is catalogued in the Transvaal Museum as Sts 71. Schepers (1950) estimated its endocranial capacity as 480 to 520 c.c., and this range of values I have employed in my tables.*

Other values have been claimed on the basis of very fragmentary remains from Sterkfontein. For example, *"Plesianthropus type 2"* was estimated at 510 to 580 c.c. by Schepers in 1946 and 520 to 540 c.c. by Schepers in 1950, whilst, by highly indirect reasoning, the cranium associated with the large mandible, Sts 7, was estimated to have a capacity of "well over 700 c.c. and perhaps more than 750 c.c." (Broom and Robinson 1948). Along with Le Gros Clark (1947, 1964) and other workers, I have not accepted these estimates in my tabulations, since the supporting evidence is not convincing.

Thus, the 4 Sterkfontein values that seem to have most evidence to support them and, accordingly, to be the more reliable ones are as follows:

Sts 60	435 c.c.
Sts 5	480 c.c.
Sts 19/58	530 c.c.
Sts 71	480 to 520 c.c.

It is stressed that these are all published data based on earlier reconstructions or, in the case of Sts 5, on an actual capacity determination. I have made no new determinations, reconstructions, or estimates on the Sterkfontein crania.†

MAKAPANSGAT. Only 1 of the approximately 40 australopithecine hominid remnants from the Makapansgat Limeworks Deposit (MLD) is suitable for making a reliable estimate of cranial capacity. The specimen known as MLD 37/38 from the pink breccia is a beautifully preserved cranium including the entire and undistorted braincase as far forward as the vicinity of the coronal suture (Dart 1962) (Figure 9). The vault is filled with a natural endocast in position. It is impossible to enucleate the endocast from the calvaria without destroying the vault-bones (parietals, temporals, and occipital). In size and shape MLD 37/38 is very similar to the Sterkfontein cranium, Sts 5. It is, however, somewhat wider, shorter, and lower than Sts 5. Dart opined, very reasonably in my view:

* The value obtained by Holloway (1970b) was smaller, namely 428 c.c.

† The values obtained by Holloway (1970b) on new reconstructions from these 4 crania are, respectively, 428, 485, 428, and 436 c.c.

17 🖋

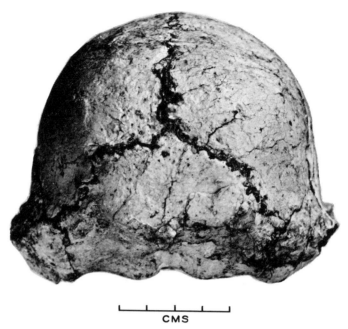

CMS

FIGURE 9: Posterior view of well-preserved, undistorted cranium of an australopithecine from Makapansgat (MLD 37/38). This specimen is estimated to have had a cranial capacity of about 480 c.c.

Whatever tendency towards increased brain size the greater parieto-temporal width [of MLD 37/38] connotes was probably completely offset by the shortening and lowering of the skull so probably the cranial capacity was no greater than that of the Sterkfontein female [Sts 5]. [Dart 1962, p. 126]

From this comparison, it seemed justified to attribute to the Makapansgat specimen the same endocranial capacity as that of Sts 5, namely 480 c.c. This value accordingly has been included in my tabulations (Tobias 1963, 1967a, 1968b).*

One other Makapansgat specimen, the original parieto-occipital piece (MLD 1), led Dart to estimate for it a capacity of no less than 650 c.c., by analogy with the claims made for the Kromdraai vault. However, it is probable that far too small a proportion of the vault of MLD 1 is preserved for the estimate to be reliable (Figure 10). Furthermore, Robinson showed

* A "quite provisional" recalculation by Holloway (1970b and personal communication) based on 4 cranial measurements and on the thickness of the first-discovered *Australopithecus* specimen from Makapansgat, MLD 1, yielded a lower value, namely 435 c.c. However, further work clearly needs to be done on the capacity of MLD 37/38.

that an alteration in the orientation of the specimen would lead to a very different interpretation as to the size of the cranial vault (Robinson 1954, p. 191). In fact, he showed that MLD 1 could be so orientated as to be "virtually indistinguishable" from that of Sts 5 from Sterkfontein. Although Robinson's diagram (ibid., Figure 5, p. 191) shows that the fit is not quite perfect, his general point seems well taken, namely that the vault of which MLD 1 was the hinder end could not have differed much in size (and capacity) from that of Sts 5, which has a capacity of 480 c.c. However, owing to the incompleteness of MLD 1, it would seem unwise at this stage to include any estimate for it in the list of fairly reliable cranial capacities.

Summary on specimens from Taung, Sterkfontein, and Makapansgat. The preceding 6 specimens—1 from Taung, 4 from Sterkfontein, and 1 from Makapansgat—have all been attributed to one species, the gracile form of australopithecine, *A. africanus* (Robinson 1954). The 6 "adult values," based on published data, are given in Table 2. In computing the

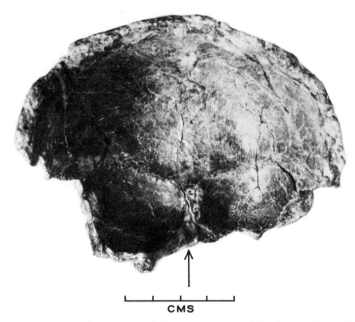

CMS

FIGURE 10: Endocranial surface of the parieto-occipital portion of an australopithecine calvaria from Makapansgat. This specimen, MLD 1, was the first hominid fragment to be recovered from the northernmost of the 5 South African australopithecine sites.

TABLE 2: *"Adult" values of cranial capacity in Australopithecus africanus* [a]	
Taung (adult value)	540 c.c.
Sts 60	435 c.c.
Sts 5	480 c.c.
Sts 71	480–520 c.c.
Sts 19/58	530 c.c.
MLD 37/38	480 c.c.
Mean ($n = 6$)	494 c.c.

[a] Based on data published by 1969.

mean for these 6 values I have used the middle value for Sts 71, namely 500 c.c. The resulting mean, 494 c.c., is lower than 2 previous estimates of the *A. africanus* mean for which I have been responsible.

In 1963, using 600 c.c. as the "adult value" for the Taung specimen, I obtained a mean for the same 6 specimens of 504 c.c. Subsequently, using the figures of Ashton and Spence (1958), I recomputed the adult value of Taung as 562 c.c. (based on a juvenile value of 520 c.c.) (Tobias 1965a). In this latest estimate I have used the same correction factor from Ashton and Spence, but I have applied it to the lower juvenile value for Taung, 500 c.c., giving the new adult estimate of 540 c.c. The effect has been a further reduction of the *A. africanus* mean from 498 (Tobias 1967a) to 494 c.c.

In 1966 Robinson stated that he had had occasion to reinvestigate the evidence relating to cranial capacity in the australopithecines. He found that 6 estimates were possible for *A. africanus*, but unfortunately he did not specify which specimens he based this statement on, nor whether they were the same 6 as those previously listed in my 1963 tabulation. Of his 6 estimates, he described 2 as very good ones and 4 as of lesser reliability. He found a mean of only 430 c.c., and the population range, based on limits of 2.5 times the standard deviation on either side of the mean, was 300 to 550 c.c. Robinson's new mean is lower than the previously accepted minimum individual value of 435 c.c. for any available australopithecine cranium! Indeed, his mean is practically the same as Holloway's minimum estimate of 428 c.c. based on new reconstructions. Presumably, Robinson has had to overthrow most of the published estimates. Unfortunately, he has not given the all-important individual data on which his new mean is based.* Even

* Holloway's (1970b) new estimates for the same 6 *A. africanus* crania as have been used by myself give a mean capacity of 442 c.c., which is not quite as low as Robinson's new estimate but is still appreciably lower than the previous mean of 494 c.c. The standard deviation for this sample of 6 gracile australopithecine capacities is estimated by Holloway as 21.59 c.c., giving a coefficient of variation of 4.88 per cent. Two of Holloway's reestimates are less reliable or definitive than the others, namely those for Sts 19 and for MLD 37/38, which are, respectively, 94 c.c. and 45 c.c. less than the values listed above by myself. If we disregard the admittedly

if he has not made allowances for the childhood status of the Taung skull, this omission would lower the mean by only about 7 c.c.

The robust australopithecines

SWARTKRANS AND KROMDRAAI. Although a large number of hominid crania has been recovered from Swartkrans, not one of them is sufficiently complete and undistorted to have permitted an accurate estimate to be made of the endocranial capacity. True, statements about the capacity of the Swartkrans (SK) specimens are not wanting in the literature.

Broom and Robinson (1952) recorded estimates for 2 child crania from Swartkrans; the first was 700 c.c. (for an adolescent, supposed female) and the other 750 to 800 c.c. (for a six- to seven-year-old, presumed male). For 3 adult crania from Swartkrans the same authors had provided estimates of about 750 (SK 48), probably over 800 (SK 46), and probably over 1000 c.c., respectively. Robinson stated that a juvenile from Swartkrans had a braincase length 20 to 25 mm. greater than that of the Taung child and a breadth proportionately greater. He claimed, in consequence, "From this and the adult crania in our possession it seems that the general order of brain size of the adult *P. crassidens* * is comparable with that of the smaller specimens of *Pithecanthropus*—roughly 800 cm.³" (Robinson 1952, p. 197). All of the foregoing estimates were based on crushed, damaged, and incomplete specimens, not one of which allowed a precise estimate to be made. Consequently, few or no workers have accepted these claims for the capacity of the Swartkrans specimens. Nevertheless, weakly based as these guesses were, it had become accepted by a number of workers that the cranial capacity of *A. robustus* (= *Paranthropus*) was greater than that of the gracile *A. africanus*. This is implied, for instance, by Le Gros Clark in his discussion on cranial capacity. He states:

The Swartkrans skulls and jaws are considerably larger than those found at Sterkfontein, but, unfortunately, none of the calvariae are sufficiently well preserved to permit accurate estimates of cranial capacity. [Le Gros Clark 1964, p. 133]

The impression that the robust australopithecine had a larger cranial capacity than the gracile was supported by the estimate for the original

most provisional of Holloway's reestimates, that for MLD 37/38, and use the previously accepted value of 480 c.c., together with Holloway's new figures for the other 5 crania, this still gives a sample mean of 450 c.c., an estimate of the standard deviation, derived from the sample range, of 22.49 c.c., and a coefficient of variation of 5.00 per cent.

* His name, at that time, for the robust australopithecine from Swartkrans.

Kromdraai cranium. Despite the fact that the vault is represented by little more than the squamous portion of the left temporal bone, the greater wing of the left sphenoid, the lower part of the left parietal, and part of the left side of the occipital bone, Schepers made a number of attempts at reconstruction. These studies yielded values ranging from 575 to 680 c.c., "650 c.c. representing the average" (Schepers 1946, p. 238). The figure 650 was cited by Broom and Robinson in 1948, by Schepers in 1950, and by Dart in 1956. However, as Le Gros Clark pointed out,

The remains of the skull found at Kromdraai do not permit of even an approximate estimation of cranial capacity, but it is at least apparent from the size of the endocranial casts of the preserved temporal and cerebellar regions of the cranial wall that it must have exceeded that of the Sterkfontein specimens. [Le Gros Clark 1964, p. 133]

All of the aforementioned specimens from Swartkrans and Kromdraai were so imperfect that not one of the estimates cited, ranging from 650 to "probably over 1000," has gained general acceptance, and none of them has been included in my tabulations (Tobias 1963, 1967a, 1968b).

The first convincing evidence that robust australopithecines might have had cranial capacities of the same order of magnitude as the gracile ones was provided by the hyper-robust specimen, Olduvai hominid (Old. Hom.) 5 from Olduvai, found by Dr. Mary Leakey in July 1959. The specimen is discussed in the ensuing section. Its capacity was no larger than that of some of the larger-brained of the *A. africanus* sample (530 c.c., Tobias 1963).

This specimen brought a clear demonstration that, if the estimates of capacity of the larger-brained skulls of *A. africanus* were accurate, then the cheek-teeth, jaws, and bony buttresses of the masticatory apparatus in the robust australopithecines were disproportionately large, *without any accompanying enlargement of the brain* (Tobias 1967a, p. 80). A year after the discovery of the Olduvai specimen Robinson, in an address to the South African Association for the Advancement of Science in July 1960, revised his estimate of the cranial capacity of the robust australopithecines, lowering the high values quoted above to a modest 450 to 550 c.c.—the same order of size as obtains in the gracile *A. africanus* (Robinson 1961). He said then of the australopithecines in general, "The endocranial volume appears to be only about 500 cm.^{3}—I know of no sound evidence at present indicating a brain significantly larger than this. The range is evidently about

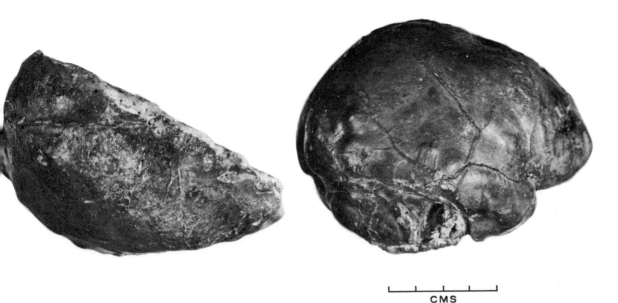

CMS

FIGURE 11: Norma verticalis (*left*) and norma lateralis (*right*) of the new endocranial cast (SK 1585) of a hominid from Swartkrans. This is the most perfectly preserved endocast yet found at any of the South African sites that have yielded the robust australopithecine (*Australopithecus robustus*); however, another hominid has been identified from the same site, namely a member of the genus *Homo* (originally called *Telanthropus*). The photographs of the new endocast were generously supplied by Dr. C. K. Brain, Director of the Transvaal Museum, and discoverer of the specimen.

450 to 550 cm.^{3}" In his definition of *Paranthropus* (1962b, p. 138) he cited "an endocranial volume of the order of 450 to 550 cm.^{3}" as one of its features.

Thus, until very recently, no specimen provided clearcut evidence on the cranial capacity of the South African robust form. On 17 January 1966, C. K. Brain, in a new excavation at Swartkrans, found a superbly preserved hominid endocranial cast, SK 1585 (1968a, 1969) (Figure 11). He has kindly permitted me to quote his as yet unpublished estimate of its capacity, namely 475 c.c. Holloway has made an independent study and reconstruction of the missing parts of the endocast, from which he finds a higher value, namely 530 c.c. (the same value as that for the Olduvai specimen, Old. Hom. 5). The difference between the 2 estimates is appreciable. Dr.

Brain has generously invited me to make a definitive study of the specimen in question, but at the time of writing I have not yet made this study. Nor have I yet made a third and independent estimation of the capacity. For the moment, it would seem to be safest to choose an intermediate value, namely 500 c.c., between Brain's and Holloway's estimates as an approximation to the total capacity of the Swartkrans specimen.

The value of 500 c.c. (or even that of 530 c.c. and a fortiori of 475 c.c.) lies within the sample range given by me for the gracile australopithecines (435 to 540 c.c.). This is the first and thus far the only reliable estimate of the cranial capacity from a South African site yielding robust australopithecines. However, it must not be overlooked that the same site, Swartkrans, has yielded a second hominid, which has been identified as a member of the genus *Homo* and was originally called *Telanthropus*. To which of the 2 Swartkrans hominids the new endocast belongs must for the time being remain an open question, although it is tempting to infer that its relatively small volume would tend to align it with *Australopithecus* rather than with *Homo*.

OLDUVAI. The hominid cranium found in the lower part of Bed I, Olduvai Gorge, has been described as a hyper-robust australopithecine, *A. boisei* (Tobias 1967a), formerly designated *Zinjanthropus* (Leakey 1959) (Figure 12). No natural endocast was found with the cranial remains of this Old. Hom. 5 specimen. However, enough of the endocranial surface of the calvaria was preserved to make possible the preparation of a plaster endocast (Figure 3). This was effected by me, with the invaluable expert assistance of Mr. A. R. Hughes (Supervisor of Laboratories in the Witwatersrand Department of Anatomy) and Mr. T. W. Kaufman (formerly of the staff of the same department). Approximately the posterior two-thirds of the braincase was virtually complete; likewise the calvarial parts related to the frontal poles and rostral regions. The areas between had to be reconstructed. There is little doubt as to the intervening distance because of a satisfactory approximation of the anterior and posterior calvarial parts.

On the basis cranii the gap includes the anterior part of the middle cranial fossa and most of the anterior cranial fossa. Thus, the precise extent of the temporal lobes of the endocast and the exact position of the temporal poles could not be determined from the surviving cranial bones. A guide to these points is provided by the body of the sphenoid, most of

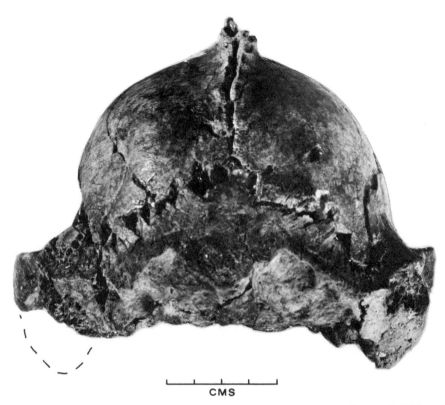

FIGURE 12: Norma occipitalis (posterior view) of the cranium of Olduvai hominid 5, the type specimen of *Australopithecus boisei*. Its artificial endocast made by me, assisted by A. R. Hughes and T. W. Kaufman, is shown in Figure 3. The volume of the total endocast has been determined as 530 c.c.

which is present as far forward as the posterior half or more of the hypophyseal fossa on its dorsum, whilst ventrally a substantial part of the vomer articulates with the sphenoid rostrum. In higher Primates the medial aspect of the temporal poles abuts close to the body of the sphenoid.

Available for comparison was a large collection of plaster endocranial casts of gorilla, chimpanzee, orangutan, cercopithecoids, *Homo erectus* and other fossil hominines, and modern man, as well as australopithecine natural endocasts, and plaster endocasts of those australopithecines for which no natural endocast had formed or been found.

Under such circumstances, it is felt that the plaster endocast of Old. Hom. 5 cannot be far from the mark and cannot deviate volumetrically from the true cranial capacity by more than perhaps 10 to 20 c.c. in either direction.

The endocast was varnished and its volume determined by displacement of water. In 7 determinations the displaced water was measured by volume and in 3 further determinations by weight. The mean of the first 7 estimations was 529.7 c.c.; the mean of the next 3 estimations was 528.1 c.c.; and the overall mean for 10 estimations was 529.2 c.c. For practical purposes, I have accepted the value of 530 c.c. (Tobias 1963, 1967a).

This Olduvai australopithecine falls somewhat short of full adulthood, the third molars being not yet in the fully erupted position of occlusion. The age of the youth may have been fifteen to sixteen years. Very little, if any, further growth of the brain occurs after this age. In modern man, for instance, brain growth is said to end at about twenty or twenty-one years of age (Marchand 1902, Pfister 1903, Zuckerman 1928), although a few workers would extend the period of growth somewhat longer (Zuckerman 1928). For chimpanzee, Zuckerman found that "there is evidence for continuation of growth into the resting stage preceding the eruption of the third molar" (1928, p. 21). Earlier (p. 17) he states, "All the evidence suggests a possible continuation of growth [in capacity of chimpanzee crania] until the stage preceding the eruption of the third molars, but there is no evidence as yet for any growth after that period." Old. Hom. 5 is precisely at the stage immediately preceding the complete eruption of the third molars.

Zuckerman's conclusions about the dental age at which growth of the cranial capacity ceases received some support from the data of Ashton and Spence (1958), although in their study all crania between the stage of eruption of the first molars and the completion of the permanent dentition were lumped into a single category.

According to Weidenreich (1941, p. 414), the cessation of actual brain growth coincides in man and pongids with the eruption of the third molar. In the light of these comparative data, since Old. Hom. 5 is almost dentally mature, the value of 530 c.c. may be accepted as the adult cranial capacity.

Thus, the value for *A. boisei* coincides with that obtained by Holloway for the Swartkrans endocast of *A. robustus* and with the capacity of the largest-brained of the 4 Sterkfontein specimens for which capacity estimates are available. It is, on the other hand, slightly bigger than the middle value for the Swartkrans specimen (500 c.c.).

TABLE 3: *Cranial capacity estimates of available sample of Australopithecus sensu lato* [a]

Specimen	Capacity (in c.c.)	Specimen	Capacity (in c.c.)
Taung (adult value)	540 (440)	Sterkfontein 71	480–520 (428)
Sterkfontein 60	435 (428)	Sts 19/58	530 (436)
Sterkfontein 5	480 (485)	MLD 37/38	480 (435)
Mean for 6 South African gracile australopithecine specimens (*A. africanus*)			494 (442)
Swartkrans (SK 1585) (*A. robustus*)	500 (530)	Olduvai (Old. Hom. 5) (*A. boisei*)	530 (530)
Australopithecinae (adult sample range) (*n* = 8)			435–540 (428–530)

[a] The values in parentheses are those of Holloway (1970b).

Estimate of population range for A. africanus

Table 3 summarizes all the data for the presently available sample of australopithecines (*n* = 8). From the *A. africanus* sample, an attempt may be made to arrive at population limits for the taxon. First, it is necessary to compute a *standard deviation* of the mean (S.D.) from this small sample. Rather than estimate this from the actual deviations from the sample mean, an estimate of the standard deviation for the population has been derived from the sample range, following Simpson, Roe, and Lewontin (1960, p. 141, Table 1a) and Lindley and Miller (1953, p. 7, Table 6). The S.D. on this basis is 41.5 c.c. (My former estimate of 47 c.c.—Tobias 1968b —was based upon a sample of 7 australopithecine estimates, including *A. boisei* of Olduvai; furthermore, as the "adult value" for Taung, I then used the figure of 562 c.c.) For comparison, Robinson's latest proposed S.D. for 6 *A. africanus* values is 50 c.c. (derived from the range quoted by him—1966, p. 958), whereas that of Holloway (1970) is only 21.59 c.c.

An estimate of the gracile australopithecine population range based on the formula, sample mean ±3 S.D., gives values of 370 to 618 c.c. when the sample mean of 494 c.c. and S.D. of 41.5 c.c. are employed.* (This contrasts

* Computed from Holloway's provisional mean of 442 c.c. and his standard deviation of 21.59, the estimated population range, based on mean ±3 S.D., is 377 to 507 c.c., that is, a remarkably similar lower limit, but an upper limit well short of the previous estimate. On a mean of 450 c.c. and S.D. of 22.49 c.c. (see footnote on page 21), the limits would be 383 to 517 c.c. However, as Holloway (1970b) has pointed out, 21.59 c.c. is an extremely small S.D. when compared with the variation of extant pongid samples: this smallness is "probably due to both the small sample size of gracile forms, and a bias introduced from using certain gracile forms to estimate the volume of others" (1970b, p. 968, note 8).

with my former estimate of 461 to 643 c.c. for *Australopithecus* sensu lato—Tobias 1968b—now hereby superseded: and with Robinson's estimate of 300 to 550 c.c. for *A. africanus*—Robinson 1966.) My latest estimate of the *A. africanus* population range is based upon a distribution about the present sample mean of 494 c.c. This would be a valid estimate if the present sample of 6 *A. africanus* capacities were drawn from the middle reaches of the population distribution. Such values as 650 c.c. for the braincase represented by the Makapansgat occipital would then be improbable.

However, through sampling bias, the present australopithecine sample may give a poor indication of the population mean. In the extreme case, if 540 c.c., the value that was estimated for the Taung adult and that forms the highest value in the sample, were also the highest value in the population, the estimated population range would be 291 to 540 c.c. Conversely, if 435 c.c., the lowest value in the sample, coincided with the lowest value in the population, the estimated population range would be 435 to 684 c.c.

It may tentatively be concluded that *if* the 6 australopithecines whose cranial capacities have been enumerated above were members of a single population, and *if* the population variability (as expressed by the range) were of the order of 6 times the estimated standard deviation, then it would be highly unlikely that any normal adult *A. africanus* cranium still to be discovered would have a capacity smaller than 291 c.c. or greater than 684 c.c.* The latter value is smaller than the smallest capacity in *H. erectus* (750 c.c.). It is smaller than 2 earlier estimates of an imaginary cerebral "Rubicon" between ape and man, that of Vallois (800 c.c.) and that of Keith (750 c.c.). Interestingly, too, the estimated upper value of 684 c.c. is exceeded by the largest capacity known in a gorilla (752 c.c.)!

We may conclude that the estimates of 1000 c.c. for the upper limits of the australopithecine cranial capacity (Broom and Robinson 1952; Dart 1956a) are excessive and highly unlikely. In a former estimate I stated that "the most generous estimate yields a maximum of 848 c.c. at the australopithecine grade of hominid organization" (Tobias 1963); but this value, which is now seen to be far too high, was based on comparison with living hominoids and not on a statistical analysis of the variance of the sample itself. The reason that comparison with values for living hominoids yields improbable results is discussed below.

The "middle reach" range of 370 to 618 c.c. is the most likely popula-

* On the basis of Holloway's (1970b) reestimates, these extreme outside limits would be of the order of 350 to 560 c.c.

tion estimate of the upper and lower limits of cranial capacity in *A. africanus*.

For the robust and hyper-robust australopithecines, the data are too scanty to permit a similar computation to be made. All that can be said at the moment is that the 2 available estimates, 500 c.c. and 530 c.c., fall within the *A. africanus* sample range and, a fortiori, within the estimated population range for *A. africanus*. Thus, as yet there is no acceptable evidence to support the idea that the robust australopithecines were significantly larger-brained than the gracile ones (Figure 13).*

ARE WE JUSTIFIED IN USING 3 S.D.S ABOVE THE SAMPLE MEAN AS THE UPPER LIMIT? For a normally distributed variate, it would seem to be perfectly reasonable to employ 3 standard deviations above and below the sample mean for estimating the limits of the population range. In fact, for many variates, palaeontologists and mammalogists are content with 2.5 S.D.s departure from the mean. Hence, in employing 3 S.D.s one might be thought to be allowing an appreciable safety margin. However, it has been questioned whether, in the instance of cranial capacity, these limits do provide a realistic picture of the population distribution. Robinson, in particular, has questioned this assumption. He states:

The mean (cranial capacity for 6 specimens of *A. africanus*) was 430 cm.³ and the range, using limits of 2.5 times the standard deviation on either side of the mean, was 300–550 cm.³ On comparing these figures with similar ones calculated for pongids and modern man from data, based on substantial samples, provided by Ashton and Spence (1958), it became obvious to me that even limits of three times the standard deviation seriously underestimate the upper limit of the observed range for both the gorilla and man. This being the case, it is possible that the *Australopithecus* range could similarly be underestimated. Using the percentage for man as a basis for adjustment, a corrected upper value of 680 cm.³ was obtained and one of just more than 600 cm.³ on the basis of the gorilla discrepancy. [Robinson 1966, p. 958]

Unfortunately, once again Robinson has not given the essential data on which he has based these computations. One would wish to know what value he employed for the S.D. of man and gorilla; what upper limit he employed for the ranges for man and gorilla in terms of number of cubic

---

* Based on Holloway's (1970b) estimates, the robust australopithecines with a mean of 530 c.c. (*n* = 2) are significantly greater in capacity than the gracile australopithecines with a mean of 442 c.c. (*n* = 6).

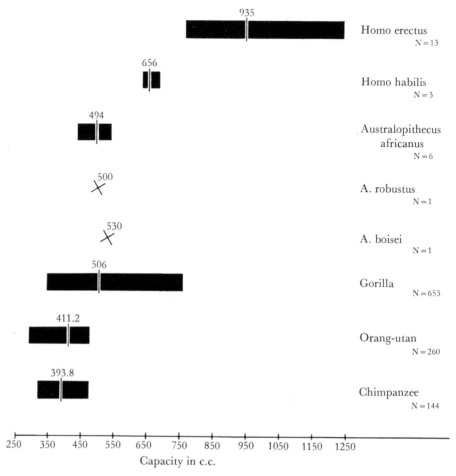

FIGURE 13: The cranial capacities of available samples of fossil hominids compared with those of extant great apes. The sample mean is indicated in each instance by a narrow vertical line. No attempt has been made in this diagram to separate the sample for each hominoid into male and female subsamples.

centimeters and, then, in terms of numbers of S.D.s departure from the sample mean. None of these data, however, has been given. Subsequently, he returned to this theme:

. . . it seems clear that variation in brain size in modern man and also the Afri-can great apes is such that the observed upper limits exceed appreciably, espe-cially in man, the traditional limit set by three times the standard deviation above the mean calculated from samples of substantial size. [Robinson 1968, p. 171]

He continues by speculating on the possibility that in *Australopithecus,* too, the upper limits of the range of cranial capacities might have exceeded "appreciably" a value based on the mean $+$ 3 S.D.s.

Still fewer supporting data are given in this statement, and it is interesting to note that where previously he had referred only to man and gorilla as having what he considered extraordinarily high upper limits he now speaks of man and "the African great apes," thereby presumably including chimpanzee, the other African great ape.

Robinson thus proposes to introduce a correction factor, and, from the earlier reference cited (p. 29), he bases this correction on the range of variation found in gorilla and modern human cranial capacities. The validity of his inference depends in large measure on 3 factors: how he has derived his interracial mean and standard deviation for modern man and gorilla; whether he has used appropriately weighted estimates of these 2 statistics; and the validity of his choice of these 2 hominoids, namely man and gorilla, as the basis for analogy.

Unfortunately, neither of the first 2 issues is dealt with, and no evidence is cited in support of the third proposition—the validity of choosing man and gorilla, but not apparently chimpanzee or orangutan.

This last point would seem to be the most serious criticism of the correction Robinson has proposed to make. Since he has made no attempt to justify his choice of man and gorilla as the 2 living hominoid taxa from which to derive his correction factor, it has proved necessary to examine this question more closely. His proposed new australopithecine mean of 430 c.c. is the figure on which he has based his computations. Yet this figure of 430 c.c. is far closer to the means for orangutan (411.2 c.c. for a combined sample of 260 males and females) and for chimpanzee (393.8 c.c. for a combined sample of 144 males and females), than it is to the means for gorilla (498.3 c.c. for a combined sample of 533 males and females; or 506 c.c. for 653 males) or for modern man (interracial mean of 1334 c.c. based on Bailey and von Bonin 1951). Despite this greater proximity of his estimate of the australopithecine mean to the means for chimpanzee and orangutan, Robinson has chosen the 2 taxa that, by his analysis, have means further removed from his estimate for *Australopithecus africanus.* It would seem to be implied that *A. africanus* is of a comparable order of variability, with comparable occasional high values, to man and gorilla.

A closer look at the distributions of the available samples of modern hominoid cranial capacities has revealed certain peculiarities (Tobias 1968b) that may seriously affect the question of selecting one or another taxon for analogy with *A. africanus*.

 # THE CRANIAL CAPACITY
OF MODERN HOMINOIDS

Means and ranges

Tables 4 to 7 summarize virtually all the available data for living hominoids. For each species, the sample size, the sample range, and the sample mean are given.

GIBBONS AND SIAMANGS. The values for the hylobatines (Table 4) are those of Oppenheim (1912), Schultz (1933, 1944, 1965), and Kirchner (1895). For the most part, samples for individual species and a single sex are very small. The best hylobatine series are the Chiengmai populations of *Hylobates lar,* of which Schultz (1944, 1965) obtained no fewer than 95 males and 86 females. Kirchner's series of *H. concolor* capacities, though large ($n = 63$), is based on combined male and female data, as cited by Selenka (1898) and Schultz (1933). Unfortunately, I did not have access to the original 1895 doctoral thesis of Kirchner, from which Selenka and Schultz quoted his data. Where combined sex data (or data for unsexed material) for any one species are cited in the literature, I have included these in the Table, for example, Schultz's (1933) data for 10 male + female *H. klossii,* which would appear to be the only data available for this species. However, the figures cited by Vallois (1954) for *Hylobates* and for *Symphalangus* have not been included, as they comprise pooled data not only for both sexes, but also for a number of species.

For the siamang data in Table 4 I have pooled individual figures given by Oppenheim (1912) with the data of Schultz (1933) to provide modest samples of 23 male and 17 female capacities. The procedure of pooling data, though sanctified by long usage, is of course liable to introduce errors based on (a) possible geographical or racial differences in mean capacity, and (b) differences in filling material and technique employed by different workers. However, where the individual samples are small, the error introduced by pooling is probably no greater than the error which might be imported by using such small samples to draw conclusions about the population mean.

The limited data available suggest that siamangs have mean capacities about 25 per cent greater than do gibbons. Among the gibbons, male means for most species are clustered around 100 to 104 c.c., though it seems that *H. klossii* may have a somewhat lower capacity, as Schultz (1933) stressed.

CHIMPANZEES. Table 5 gives available data for both species of chimpanzee, *Pan troglodytes* being well represented, and *P. paniscus* poorly so. Data are given for individual series and pooled totals for each sex, and for combined male and female totals. The combined-sex data are included purposefully, partly because several such series are available in the literature, and partly because various workers had used the distribution characteristics of such mixed samples of extant hominoids to make inferences about the distribution of capacities among fossil taxa. It was therefore important to study the differences in distribution between unisexual and bisexual samples.

The overall male mean is about 400 c.c. in *P. troglodytes* and the female mean close to 375 c.c. Technical and, possibly, population differences are suggested by the rather striking range of sample means. For males, these range from as low as 381 c.c. for Schultz's (1965) large series to 420 c.c. for Selenka's (1898) series. A similarly large fluctuation is evident among females, the sample means ranging from Schultz's low figure of 350 c.c. to Selenka's high mean of 390 c.c. For both sexes, Zuckerman's (1928) means are close to midway between Schultz's and Selenka's, while the data of Ashton and Spence (1958) are in each sex one quarter of the distance from the top of the range of means (that is, about midway between Zuckerman's and Selenka's means).

These regularities are reflected in a fairly constant sex ratio as determined by the various workers. Thus, the female mean expressed as a percentage of the male mean is 92.9 (Selenka), 92.7 (Ashton and Spence), 91.8 (Schultz), and 91.6 (Zuckerman). Only Oppenheim's male and female means are somewhat inconsistent, giving a sex ratio of 96.2 per cent. The sex ratio of the pooled means (including Oppenheim's) is 93.1 per cent.

TABLE 4: *Cranial capacity in living adult hylobatines*

Series	Size of sample	Sample range (in c.c.)	Sample mean (in c.c.)	Reference
GIBBONS				
Hylobates lar				
Males	13	85–114	98.9	After Schultz 1933
Males (Chiengmai)	95	89–125	104.0	Schultz 1944
Females	7	84–118	97.6	After Schultz 1933
Females (Chiengmai)	85	82–116	100.9	Schultz 1944
Females (Chiengmai)	86	82–116	101.0	Schultz 1965
Combined males and females	4	70–130	94.7	Oppenheim 1912
Hylobates "entelloides"				
Combined males and females	4	89–100	94.7	Oppenheim 1912
Hylobates agilis				
Males	8	87–111	98.7	Schultz 1933
Females	5	86–103	92.0	Schultz 1933
Combined males and females	8	81–120	103.1	Oppenheim 1912
Combined males and females	21	81–120	98.8	Schultz 1933 (based on Oppenheim 1912 and Schultz 1933)
Hylobates pileatus				
Males	2	99–104	101.5	After Schultz 1933
Females	7	81–104	91.4	After Schultz 1933
Combined males and females	9	81–104	93.7	Schultz 1933

	N	Range	Mean	Source
Hylobates concolor				
Males	4	85–136	104.3	After Schultz 1933
Females	2	93–97	95.0	After Schultz 1933
Combined males and females	63	82–130	?	Kirchner 1895 (cited by Selenka 1898)
Combined males and females	6	85–136	101.2	Schultz 1933
Combined males and females	(69)	82–136	(101.2)	Schultz 1933
Hylobates cinereus (= "leuciscus" of Oppenheim 1912)				
Males	2	103–104	103.5	After Schultz 1933
Females	4	94–115	104.0	After Schultz 1933
Combined males and females	4	80–90	86.6	Schultz 1933 (after Oppenheim 1912)
Combined males and females	10	80–115	96.9	Schultz 1933
Hylobates hoolock				
Combined males and females	3	93–100	96.0	Schultz 1933
Hylobates klossii				
Combined males and females	10	78–103	87.1	Schultz 1933
SIAMANGS				
Symphalangus syndactylus				
Males	23	100–150	125.8	This study (based on Oppenheim 1912 and Schultz 1933)
Females	17	105–152	122.8	This study (based on Oppenheim 1912 and Schultz 1933)
Combined males and females	40	100–152	124.6	Schultz 1933

35

TABLE 5: *Cranial capacity in living adult hominoids: chimpanzee*

Series	Size of sample	Sample range (in c.c.)	Sample mean (in c.c.)	Reference
Pan troglodytes				
Males	24	350–480	420.0	Selenka 1899
Males	? [a]	350–470	404.3	Oppenheim 1911–1912
Males	34	325–500	399.5	Zuckerman 1928
Males	33	Not stated	410.0	Ashton and Spence 1958
Males	56	292–454	381.0	Schultz 1965
Total pooled males	163 [b]	292–500 [c]	398.5	This study
Females	26	320–450	390.0	Selenka 1899
Females	? [a]	350–440	388.8	Oppenheim 1911–1912
Females	27	290–455	365.8	Zuckerman 1928
Females	78	Not stated	380.0	Ashton and Spence 1958
Females	57	282–415	350.0	Schultz 1965
Total pooled females	200 [b]	282–460 [c]	371.1	This study
Combined males and females	61	290–500	384.5	Zuckerman 1928
Combined males and females	144	320–480	393.8	Vallois 1954
Combined males and females	111	Not stated	390.0	Ashton and Spence 1958
Combined males and females	363	282–500	383.4	This study
Pan paniscus				
Males	6	334–381	356.0	Schultz 1965
Females	5	275–358	329.0	Schultz 1965

[a] Oppenheim (1911–1912) gave the total for both sexes combined as 40, but she did not give the sexual or age breakdown of this figure.

[b] This total excludes Oppenheim's sample but includes several small samples culled from the literature but not listed individually here.

[c] The range for the pooled sample assumes that the extreme values for the sample of Ashton and Spence do not lie outside the limiting values of the other samples. The female upper limiting value (460 c.c.) is the capacity of a cranium studied by T. L. W. Bischoff (1867) cited by Zuckerman (1928).

The miniscule samples of *P. paniscus* suggest a mean capacity about 10 per cent lower than that of *P. troglodytes* for each sex.

ORANGUTANS. Table 6 gives data for 5 main series of each sex, as well as pooled and combined-sex data. Once again, there is an impressive range of sample means, that for males extending from 395 c.c. (Oppenheim 1911–1912) to 455 c.c. (Selenka 1898, 1899), whilst that for females stretches from 338 c.c. (Schultz 1965) to 390 c.c. (Selenka 1898, 1899; Gaul 1933). The size of the extreme range of sample means is thus 50 to 60 c.c. That there are population differences in mean capacity within *Pongo pygmaeus* is suggested by the work of Selenka and of Gaul: this factor may account for the appreciably greater range of sample means in the orangutan than in the chimpanzee, although their overall mean capacities are close. Sexual dimorphism is greater among the orangs than among the chimpanzees. Thus, while the means of the total pooled male series are 434.4 c.c. for orang and 398.5 c.c. for chimpanzee, the female means are practically the same in the 2 species, being 374.5 c.c. in orang and 371.1 c.c. in chimpanzee, for comparably large samples. The sex ratio for the pooled samples of orang is as low as 86.2 per cent, as compared with 93.1 per cent in chimpanzee. However, there are wide fluctuations among the results of various workers: for individual series, the sex ratios are 90.5 (Oppenheim), 89.8 (Gaul), 89.2 (Ashton and Spence), 85.7 (Selenka), and 81.3 (Schultz).

GORILLAS. In Table 7 are given available data on gorillas. For 8 male series the sample means range from 497 to 551 c.c.: the size of the extreme range of sample means (54 c.c.) is thus rather less than that for male orangutan (60 c.c.). For female gorilla the sample means cluster more closely, between 442 and 478 c.c., an extreme range of only 36 c.c., whereas the range for female orangutan is 52 c.c. It should be noted, however, that 4 out of the 8 female gorilla samples are extremely small (5 to 12 crania). If we confine our attention to the remaining 4 samples, those of Selenka (1899), Randall (1943–1944), Ashton and Spence (1958), and Schultz (1965), our sample means range only from 443 to 461 c.c. Thus, both for male and female gorilla the range of sample means is absolutely smaller than the range for orangutan, despite the 80 to 100 c.c. by which gorilla means exceed orang means. This might suggest that, if technical and sampling errors are not to blame, intraspecific diversification of mean endocranial capacity is less among gorilla than among orangutan.

TABLE 6: *Cranial capacity in living adult hominoids: orangutan*

Series	Size of sample	Sample range (in c.c.)	Sample mean (in c.c.)	Reference
Males	ca. 80	360–530	455.0	Selenka 1898, 1899
Males	?[a]	320–480	395.0	Oppenheim 1911–1912
Males	36	343–523	434.1	Gaul 1933
Males	30	Not stated	415.0	Ashton and Spence 1958
Males	57	334–502	416.0	Schultz 1965
Total pooled males	203[b]	320–540[c]	434.4	This study[d]
Females	ca. 70	300–490	390.0	Selenka 1898, 1899
Females	?[a]	300–390	357.6	Oppenheim 1911–1912
Females	59	304–494	389.8	Gaul 1933
Females	18	Not stated	370.0	Ashton and Spence 1958
Females	52	276–425	338.0	Schultz 1965
Total pooled females	199[b]	276–494[c]	374.5	This study
Combined males and females	48	Not stated	400.0	Ashton and Spence 1958
Combined males and females	260	295–475	411.2	Vallois 1954
Combined males and females	402	276–540	404.8	This study[d]

[a] Oppenheim (1911–1912) gave the combined-sex total as 43 but did not give the sexual or age breakdown of the sample.

[b] This total excludes Oppenheim's series.

[c] The range for these pooled samples assumes that the observed range of Ashton and Spence is wholly encompassed by the limiting values of the combined remaining samples.

[d] Bischoff (1867) found a capacity of 575 c.c. in a "giant" orangutan of Borneo (Novara Expedition). This cranium is reported to have had no sagittal crest (quoted by Oppenheim 1912, p. 86).

TABLE 7: *Cranial capacity in living adult hominoids: gorilla*

Series	Size of sample	Sample range (in c.c.)	Sample mean (in c.c.)	Reference
Males	13	425–573	497.0	Keith 1895
Males	50	420–590	510.0	Selenka 1899
Males	22	420–585	505.4	Oppenheim 1911–1912
Males	26 [a]	450–655	550.6	Hagedoorn 1924, 1926; Bolk 1925
Males	23	440–652	513.0	Harris 1926
Males	133	420–685	543.0	Randall 1943–1944
Males	63	Not stated	550.0	Ashton and Spence 1958
Males	72	412–752	535.0	Schultz 1965
Total pooled males (1961)	400 [b]	420–752 [c]	534.8	Schultz 1962
Total pooled males (1971)	414 [b]	412–752 [c]	534.6	This study
Females	7	393–496	450.0	Keith 1895
Females	48	380–530	450.0	Selenka 1899
Females	5	370–555	475.0	Oppenheim 1911–1912
Females	12	390–595	478.0	Hagedoorn 1924, 1926; Bolk 1925
Females	11	415–475	442.0	Harris 1926
Females	78	340–580	461.0	Randall 1943–1944
Females	50	Not stated	460.0	Ashton and Spence 1958
Females	43	350–523	443.0	Schultz 1965
Total pooled females	254	340–595 [c]	455.6	This study
Combined males and females	532	340–685	497.8	Vallois 1954
Combined males and females	653	340–752	506.0	Tobias 1967a
Combined males and females	668	340–752	504.6	This study

[a] Bolk (1925) cited n as 27 and $\bar{x}$ as 550 c.c. for Hagedoorn's (1924, 1926) gorilla data; we have used Hagedoorn's 1926 figures of 26 and 551 c.c. (550.6 c.c.).

[b] These pooled totals include several small samples culled from the literature but not listed individually here.

[c] The ranges for these pooled samples assume that the unstated observed ranges of Ashton and Spence are wholly encompassed within the limiting values of the combined remaining samples.

The ratio of the total pooled female mean to the total pooled male mean is 85.2 per cent, very similar to that for the pooled orangutan series (86.2 per cent). Again, there is a fairly wide spread of sample sex ratios, the values for which are 88.2 (Selenka), 84.9 (Randall), 83.6 (Ashton and Spence), and 82.8 (Schultz). The series of the other 4 workers cited in Table 7 are excluded from this comparison as the size of the female sample in each instance is too small.

The mean for 414 pooled male gorillas is exactly 100 c.c. greater than that for 203 pooled male orangutans (534.6 c.c. against 434.4 c.c.). In the female series the pooled gorilla mean (455.6 c.c.) exceeds the pooled orangutan mean (374.5 c.c.) by 81.1 c.c.

Schultz (1962) published a mean for 58 West African male gorilla crania, the capacities ranging from 423 to 752 c.c. with a mean of 536.1 c.c. These data are not cited separately in Table 7, as the 58 crania are included in Schultz's (1965) series of 72 male gorilla crania.

The value of 752 c.c. is the only gorilla capacity or ape capacity ever to have been measured in excess of 700 c.c. Schultz (1962) tells us that he measured the capacity of this cranium (No. 6841) extremely carefully, 4 times, with practically the same result. He made a meticulous search for signs of pathology but concluded that the animal was normal. The cranium belonged to a young adult male animal that had been shot in the wild on the northeastern frontier of Spanish Guinea in 1960.

This maximum capacity of 752 c.c. is exceptional, exceeding the previous gorilla maxima of 605 c.c. (Gyldenstolpe 1928), 623 c.c. (Weidenreich 1943), 642 c.c. (Harris 1926), 655 c.c. (Hagedoorn 1926), and 685 c.c. (Randall 1943–1944).

SUMMATION ON MEAN CRANIAL CAPACITIES. Table 8 is a brief summary of mean cranial capacities in living hominoids.

TABLE 8: *Summary of mean cranial capacities in living male and female hominoids: latest pooled data (in c.c.)*

	Males	*Females*
Gibbon (*H. lar*)	104.0 (*n* = 95)	100.9 (*n* = 85)
Siamang (*S. syndactylus*)	125.8 (*n* = 23)	122.8 (*n* = 17)
Chimpanzee (*Pan troglodytes*)	398.5 (*n* = 163)	371.1 (*n* = 200)
Orangutan (*Pongo pygmaeus*)	434.4 (*n* = 203)	374.5 (*n* = 199)
Gorilla (*G. gorilla*)	534.6 (*n* = 414)	455.6 (*n* = 254)

MATERIAL AND METHODS. In Table 9 are cited data bearing on the variability of each sample, namely the *extreme range* (or the difference between the maximum and minimum values of each sample), the estimated *standard deviation* of the mean, and the estimated *coefficient of variation* (*V*) of the sample. Similar parameters are given for pooled one-sex samples and for combined-sex series. Some of the standard deviations are given by the authors themselves, notably Randall (1943–1944), Ashton (1950), and Ashton and Spence (1958): these S.D.s are marked with a superscript *a* in Table 9. In some other published works the original raw data are listed, as by Hagedoorn (1926), Schultz (1933), and Gaul (1933); whilst Dr. Adolph Schultz generously sent me his unpublished raw data on his 95 male and 85 female capacities of *H. lar* crania from the Chiengmai District of northern Thailand. In these instances my research assistants, Miss C. J. Orkin and C. Block, computed the S.D. directly from the original data. Standard deviations obtained in this way are marked with an *a* in Table 9.

In most studies, however, the mean and the sample range are given but not the S.D. or the raw data. To compute the S.D. of the series, as well as of the pooled and combined-sex samples, we have resorted to the relationship for normally distributed variables between the sample frequency (*n*), the mean observed range, and the standard deviation. These relationships are tabulated, for example, by Simpson, Roe, and Lewontin (1960, p. 141, Table 1) and by Lindley and Miller (1953, p. 7, Table 6). Briefly, for a population that is normally distributed, the mean observed range is 6 times σ when $n = 442$, and 6.48 times σ when the sample is 1000. For smaller samples, the observed range is, of course, less adequate as an estimate of the population range: when $n = 100$, the mean observed range is only 5.02 times σ; when $n = 50$, the value is 4.50; when $n = 20$, it is 3.74; when $n = 10$, it is 3.08. Thus, while the observed range is not really an adequate substitute for the S.D. in most instances, it can be used for a rough estimation of σ, where more accuracy is not required, or where no alternative method of computing the S.D. is available, as when the raw data are not given. Accordingly, where the S.D. has not been given in a publication, or where the individual data are not listed, an estimate of the standard deviation has been made by dividing the differences between the maximum and minimum values (that is, the size of the extreme range) by the values given

41 ✗

TABLE 9: *The variability of hominoid cranial capacities*

Species and series	Size of sample	Sample mean (in c.c.)	Extreme range (observed size) of range (in c.c.)	S.D. of mean (in c.c.)	Estimated coefficient of variation (per cent)	Reference
GIBBON (*Hylobates lar*)						
Males	95	104.0	36	7.51 [a] / 7.23 [b]	7.22	Schultz 1944
Females	85	100.9	34	7.81 [a] / 6.94 [b]	7.69	Schultz 1944
GIBBON (*Hylobates agilis*)						
Combined males and females	21	98.8	39	10.32 [b]	10.45	Schultz 1933 (based on Oppenheim 1912 and Schultz 1933)
SIAMANG (*Symphalangus syndactylus*)						
Males	23	125.8	50	12.95 [b]	10.29	This study (based on Oppenheim 1912 and Schultz 1933)
Females	17	122.8	47	13.09 [b]	10.66	This study (based on Oppenheim 1912 and Schultz 1933)
CHIMPANZEE (*Pan troglodytes*)						
Males	24	420.0	130	33.33 [b]	7.94	Selenka 1899
Males	34	399.5	175	40.61 [a] / 41.77 [b]	10.17	After Zuckerman 1928
Males	33	410.0	?	47.70 [a]	11.63	Ashton and Spence 1958
Males	56	381.0	162	35.29 [b]	9.26	After Schultz 1965
Total pooled males	163	398.5	208	38.88 [b]	9.76	This study
Females	26	390.0	130	32.83 [b]	8.42	After Selenka 1899
Females	27	365.8	165	33.70 [a] / 41.25 [b]	9.21	After Zuckerman 1928
Females	78	380.0	?	35.10 [a]	9.24	Ashton and Spence 1958
Females	57	350.0	133	28.85 [b]	8.24	After Schultz 1965
Total pooled females	200	371.1	178	32.42 [b]	8.74	This study
CHIMPANZEE (*Pan paniscus*)						
Males	6	356.0	47	18.58 [b]	5.22	After Schultz 1965
Females	5	329.0	83	35.62 [b]	10.83	After Schultz 1965

ORANGUTAN
(Pongo pygmaeus)

Males	ca. 80	455.0	170	35.05 [b]	7.70	Selenka 1898, 1899
Males	?	395.0	160	?	?	Oppenheim 1911–1912
Males	36	434.1	180	50.86 [a]	11.72	Gaul 1933
Males	30	415.0	?	37.60 [a]	9.06	Ashton and Spence 1958
Males	57	416.0	168	36.44 [b]	8.76	After Schultz 1965
Males	203	434.4	220	39.93 [b]	9.19	This study
Total pooled males						
Females	ca. 70	390.0	190	39.92 [b]	10.24	After Selenka 1898, 1899
Females	?	357.6	90	?	?	Oppenheim 1911–1912
Females	59	389.8	190	36.27 [a]	9.31	Gaul 1933
Females	18	370.0	Not stated	34.90 [a]	9.43	Ashton and Spence 1958
Females	52	338.0	149	32.89 [b]	9.73	After Schultz 1965
Total pooled females	199	374.5	218	39.71 [b]	10.60	This study

GORILLA
(Gorilla gorilla)

Males	50	510.0	170	37.78 [b]	7.41	After Selenka 1899
Males	22	505.4	165	43.19 [b]	8.55	After Oppenheim 1911–1912
Males	26	550.6	205	59.44 [a]	10.80	After Hagedoorn 1924, 1926 and Bolk 1925
Males	23	513.0	212	50.71 [a]	9.88	Harris 1926
Males	133	543.0	265	50.00 [b]	9.23	Randall 1943–1944
Males	63	550.0	?	61.90 [a]	11.25	Ashton and Spence 1958
Males	72	535.0	340	71.13 [b]	13.30	After Schultz 1965
Total pooled males (1961)	400	534.8	332	55.89 [b]	10.45	After Schultz 1962
Total pooled males (1971)	414	534.6	340	57.05 [b]	10.67	This study
Females	48	450.0	150	33.56 [b]	7.46	After Selenka 1899
Females	78	461.0	240	47.70 [a]	10.34	Randall 1943–1944
Females	50	460.0	?	35.20 [a]	7.65	Ashton and Spence 1958
Females	43	443.0	173	39.41 [b]	8.90	After Schultz 1965
Total pooled females (1971)	254	455.6	255	45.13 [b]	9.91	This study
Combined males and females (1954)	532	497.8	345	56.46 [b]	11.34	After Vallois 1954
Combined males and females (1967)	653	506.0	412	66.03 [b]	13.05	After Tobias 1967a
Combined males and females (1971)	668	504.6	412	65.92 [b]	13.06	This study

MODERN MAN
(Homo sapiens)

Males	1000s	1345.0	1100–1300	ca. 169.00 [b]	12.57	This study (after many earlier studies)
				–ca. 200.00 [b]	–14.87	

for the quotient mean observed range/σ for various sizes of n. The approximate S.D.s obtained in this way are marked in Table 9 by a superscript b.

In several instances the S.D. has been computed both directly and from the range for a given sample, in order to compare the results. For fairly large samples the 2 values approximate moderately well: for example, for 95 male *H. lar,* the values obtained are 7.51 (from the deviations) and 7.23 (from the range). For 85 female *H. lar* the 2 estimates are 7.81 and 6.94, respectively. With smaller samples, however, the discrepancy is larger: for 34 male chimpanzees, the estimates are 40.61 and 41.77 c.c., whilst for 27 female chimpanzees, the estimates are 33.70 and 41.25 c.c. In the case of these 4 series, only the S.D. derived from the actual deviations has been used in the later estimates of skewing (Table 12).

The standard deviation estimated by either method is then expressed as a percentage of the sample mean to give the coefficient of variation (V).

VARIABILITY: RESULTS ON LIVING HOMINOIDS. Among the different samples of hominoid cranial capacities cited, V varies widely. For single sex samples, where n is reasonably large, the lowest value of V is 7.22 per cent (for 95 male *H. lar*), while the highest value, excluding modern man, is 13.30 per cent (for 72 male gorilla).

In the chimpanzee series, V for males varies from 7.94 to 11.63 per cent, the figure for 163 total pooled males being 9.76 per cent. Among female chimpanzees, V varies from 8.24 to 9.24 per cent, the figure for 200 pooled females being 8.74 per cent. Thus, while considerable *variability of variability* obtains among various samples of chimpanzees, the overall impression is that male capacities are somewhat more variable than female.

For male orangutan, V ranges from 7.70 to 11.72 per cent, the value for 203 pooled males being 9.19 per cent. Among females, the values of V stretch from 9.31 to 10.24 per cent, whilst the value for 199 pooled females is 10.60

NOTES TO TABLE 9:

[a] Determined from actual deviations by Ashton (1950) after Zuckerman (1928), Ashton and Spence (1958), Randall (1943–1944), and by my research assistants, Miss C. J. Orkin and Mr. C. Block.

[b] Estimated by Miss C. J. Orkin and myself from the sample range, by the use of a table of relationships between the sample frequency, the mean observed range, and the standard deviation (Simpson, Roe, and Lewontin 1960, p. 141, Table 1).

per cent. It would appear from these figures that female orang capacities are somewhat more variable than those of males.

Among gorillas, V for male capacities ranges from 7.41 to 13.30 per cent, the values for 414 pooled males being 10.67 per cent. Corresponding figures for female gorillas are 7.46 to 10.34 per cent, with a value of 9.91 for 254 pooled females.

In modern man, variability is high, with an estimated V of 12.57 to 14.87 per cent for a male sample.

Hence, in general the cranial capacity tends to be more variable the bigger it is: V for male gorilla, orangutan, and chimpanzee being 10.67, 9.19 and 9.76 per cent, respectively. Among females, the same relationship holds for gorillas and chimpanzees, with Vs of 9.91 and 8.74, respectively; but the female orangs seem to be rather anomalously variable with a V of 10.60.

ON THE USE OF COMBINED-SEX SAMPLES. Several students have made use of Vallois's (1954) figures: these, it should be stressed, are entirely of combined-sex samples. For such samples, V ranges from 7.71 to 13.06 per cent, leaving aside the figures for *Homo sapiens*. With these combined-sex samples, the 3 great apes sort themselves even more clearly: the values of V for mean cranial capacity of gorilla, orangutan, and chimpanzee are 13.06, 10.98, and 9.69 per cent, respectively (Table 9).

The wide range and high variability of gorilla cranial capacities may reflect, in part at least, a greater degree of sexual dimorphism in gorilla than in other anthropoid apes.

SEXUAL DIMORPHISM OF HOMINOID CRANIAL CAPACITIES. Different degrees of sexual dimorphism of mean cranial capacity occur among the hominoids. Thus, Oppenheim (1911–1912, p. 138) cites the following figures for the mean capacity of females expressed as a percentage of the mean capacity of males: gibbon 98, chimpanzee 95, orangutan 90, gorilla 85. Zuckerman (1928) gave 91.5 per cent as the corresponding figure for his chimpanzee series. Schultz's (1965) figures are rather similar to those of Oppenheim, except in the orangutan, for which he found a much lower percentage, that is, a much higher degree of sexual dimorphism. His figures are as follows: gibbon 97, chimpanzee 92, gorilla 83, orangutan 81. Table 10, based on the data collated in my earlier tables, gives a tolerably complete list of percentage ratios of adult female means to adult male means.

TABLE 10: *Sexual dimorphism of hominoid cranial capacity*
(*adult female mean expressed as a percentage of adult male mean*)

Species	Percentage	Source of data
Siamang (*S. syndactylus*)	97.6	This study, after Oppenheim and Schultz
Gibbon (*H. lar*)	97.0	Schultz
Chimpanzee (*Pan troglodytes*)	*93.1*	This study — pooled data
	92.9	Selenka
	92.7	Ashton and Spence
	91.8	Schultz
	91.6	Zuckerman
Orangutan (*Pongo pygmaeus*)	90.5	Oppenheim
	89.8	Gaul
	89.2	Ashton and Spence
	86.2	This study — pooled data
	85.7	Selenka
	81.3	Schultz
Gorilla (*G. gorilla*)	88.2	Selenka
	85.2	This study — pooled data
	84.9	Randall
	83.6	Ashton and Spence
	82.8	Schultz

We may summarize the latest data available for sexual dimorphism of cranial capacity in the apes as follows:

Siamang	97.6
Gibbon (*H. lar*)	97.0
Chimpanzee	93.1
Orangutan	86.2
Gorilla	85.2

It is clear that modern hominoids differ appreciably in sexual dimorphism of cranial capacity. This fact is important, as several students have used combined-sex samples in their studies (for example, Vallois 1954; Dart 1956). Differing degrees of sexual dimorphism might impart varying distribution characteristics to combined-sex samples, even were the represented proportions of the 2 sexes equal. In fact, the sexual composition of the available combined-sex samples itself varies widely. Thus, the combined-sex sample of orangutan capacities, totaling 402 values, comprises virtually equal numbers of male and female capacities (203 males, 199 females). On the other hand, the combined-sex sample for gorilla, totaling 668 capacities in all, includes nearly twice as many males as females (414 males, 254 females); while the combined-sex sample for chimpanzee has a majority of females. High sexual dimorphism, together with marked inequality in the number of each of the 2 sexes in the combined sample, may well be responsible in large measure for the extremely high variability of the combined-sex sample of gorilla capacities.

However, not all the high variability of the gorilla sample is to be laid at the door of sexual dimorphism and differing sexual composition of samples. In an all-male gorilla sample, variability is smaller than in the combined-sex sample, V being 10.67 per cent in the former and 13.06 per cent in the latter. Nevertheless, even in the all-male sample of gorilla, V is definitely higher than in any of the large all-male samples of other apes. This confirms that cranial capacity in the gorilla remains very variable, even when allowance is made for the high degree of sexual dimorphism.

In contrast, the hylobatines show a much smaller degree of sexual dimorphism than the large-brained pongids. In *H. lar*, the mean capacity for adult females is 97.0 per cent of that for adult males, and in the siamang, *S. syndactylus*, the figure is 97.6 per cent. Thus, sexual dimorphism might be expected to contribute but little, if any, additional variance to a combined-sex sample of hylobatines as compared with separate male and female samples. This inference has been tested for Schultz's samples of *H. lar* and is supported by the following figures:

Males ($n = 95$)	$V = 7.22$ per cent
Females ($n = 85$)	$V = 7.69$ per cent
Combined males and females ($n = 180$)	$V = 7.62$ per cent

Irrespective of the sexual composition of the sample, the cranial capacity of *H. lar* has a moderate variability.

If we may generalize from the foregoing, it seems permissible to infer that for species with a high degree of sexual dimorphism the combining of data for both sexes does increase the variability appreciably: this is not so, however, when male and female data for species with slight sexual dimorphism are combined.

VARIABILITY IN RELATION TO MEAN CAPACITY. It has already been mentioned that, in general, V seems to be higher the bigger is the mean cranial capacity. Table 11 summarizes relevant data for adult male specimens (data for the siamang are omitted as n is only 23).

TABLE 11: *The relationship between coefficient of variability* (*V*)
and mean cranial capacity

	n	*Mean capacity* (*males*)	*V*
Gibbon (*H. lar*)	95	104.0	7.22
Chimpanzee	163	398.5	9.76
Orangutan	203	434.4	9.19
Gorilla	414	534.6	10.67
Modern man	1000s	ca. 1345.0	12.57–14.87

In relation to biological variables in general (Simpson, Roe, and Lewontin 1960, pp. 89–92), the values of *V* for gibbons, chimpanzees, and orangutans are *high,* while gorilla and man, with *V*s over 10.00, must be considered *markedly* variable.

On the available samples of capacities, living hominoids sort themselves into 2 categories, those with high variability and those with marked variability. The 2 categories coincide with a sorting based on mean capacity: the high-variability group have mean capacities for males of 435.0 c.c. and below, while the marked-variability group have mean capacities for males of 535 c.c. and over. Somewhere between 435 and 535 c.c. there would seem to be a dividing line between highly variable and markedly variable capacities in living hominoids. .

THE VARIABILITY OF CRANIAL CAPACITY IN *Australopithecus*. Where does *Australopithecus* lie? The mean capacity of *A. africanus* is 494 c.c. according to my calculation based on published estimates, 430 c.c. according to Robinson's, 442 c.c. according to Holloway's based on new estimates, and 450 c.c. based on my re-computation of Holloway's data. But the scanty data on which these means are based do not permit us to determine whether *A. africanus* belonged to the high-variability category or to the marked-variability category. Robinson's (1966) choice of gorilla and modern man as guides to the variability, and hence to the upper value, of cranial capacity in *A. africanus* is therefore seen to be rather arbitrary and, indeed, unjustified, the more so as his revised estimate of 430 c.c. for the mean capacity in *A. africanus* is almost identical with the mean capacity in orangutan, and closer to that of the chimpanzee than to those in gorilla and modern man.

The population estimate of *V* for *Australopithecus africanus*, based on an S.D. estimated from the range, gives a value of 8.4 per cent. This lies amid the values for the high-variability group. However, as Holloway has pointed out, "It makes little sense to compare . . . [coefficients of variation] and . . . [standard deviations] for large samples ($n > 100$) with those based on very small samples, for example, chimpanzee and gorilla with australopithecines . . ." (Holloway 1966a, p. 1108).

We conclude that we simply do not have enough information from which to infer whether the variation of cranial capacity in *Australopithecus* was closest to that in chimpanzee, orangutan, gorilla, or modern man. To base deductions on gorilla and modern man only would seem to imply that the cranial capacity of *A. africanus* was of a comparable high order of variability to those of man and gorilla, and similarly showed occasional very high values. Yet modern man is highly polytypic as well as polymorphic, a factor that undoubtedly accounts for much of the high (interracial) variance of many metrical traits of modern man, including cranial capacity. We have no evidence that *A. africanus* was polytypic to a similar degree. Hence, we cannot assume that a comparable degree of variation applied to this extinct group.

The skewness of the available samples of
hominoid cranial capacities

Much has been made of the maximum cranial capacity of the gorilla (752 c.c.). Yet, it is important that this solitary reading be viewed in proper perspective. Such a value has occurred only once in 668 gorilla crania for which the capacities are on record. The second largest gorilla capacity on record is as much as 67 c.c. smaller! The value of 752 c.c. exceeds the gorilla combined male and female mean of 504.6 by 3.75 S.D.s. The second highest gorilla capacity (685 c.c.) is only 2.74 S.D.s above the combined-sex mean. From what has been said above, it would be more realistic to compare the value of 752 c.c., which came from a *male* animal, with the mean (534.6 c.c.) for the total pooled *male* series ($n = 414$): 752 c.c. is 3.81 S.D.s above this mean, whilst the second largest cranial capacity (685 c.c.) is 2.64 S.D.s above the male mean.

At the other extreme, the smallest recorded adult gorilla capacity (340 c.c.) is 2.50 S.D.s below the combined-sex mean and 2.56 S.D.s below the total pooled female mean. The lowest capacity recorded for an adult *male* gorilla (412 c.c.) is 2.15 S.D.s below the total pooled male mean.

Hence, the distribution of gorilla capacities was nearly symmetrical until Schultz (1962) discovered the gorilla cranium with 752 c.c. Clearly, this single gorilla cranium has positively skewed the distribution curve.

It was this realization that led me to examine the distributions of available samples of hominoid cranial capacities for symmetry or skewness (Tobias 1968b).

Moderately asymmetrical or "skewed" distribution curves have been defined by Simpson, Roe, and Lewontin as "those in which the highest frequency is definitely not near the ends of the distribution." They continue:

> . . . skewed curves in which the right-hand limb tapers off more gradually than the left-hand limb, hence in which the class with highest frequency is below the middle of the distribution, are said to be positively skewed, or skewed to the right. Similarly, those with the left-hand limb longer and the class with highest frequency above the middle are negatively skewed, or skewed to the left. [Simpson, Roe, and Lewontin 1960, pp. 54–55]

Without access to most of the original data, it has not been possible to determine the position of the class with highest frequency (mode) in the gorilla and most other hominoid samples. Had the raw data been available, it would have been possible to use the coefficient of skewness based upon the standardized distance between the mean and mode (ibid., p. 143). Since the mode is not known for most of these hominoid samples, nor the median (from which the mode could be approximated by the formula, mode = 3 median − 2 mean), it has not proved possible to assess the *coefficient of skewness* in the present study.

Resort has been had to an alternative method that, it is suggested, yields an approximate answer to the question of how symmetrical or how skewed the distribution is. The symmetry of the distribution curve has been tested by comparing the highest with the lowest values in the sample. For each sample, the extreme values have been expressed in terms of their deviations from the mean, both in absolute units and in standardized units (deviation divided by the estimated standard deviation of the sample mean). The degree of symmetry or skewness has here been assessed by comparing the absolute and standardized deviations of the highest value with those of the lowest value and adding the algebraic sum of the two deviations (Table 12).

The data recorded by Vallois (1954) for the gibbon showed so marked a skewing as to suggest not a normal or Quetelet distribution but a J-shaped distribution. Thus, Vallois's published mean of 89.3 c.c. is only 2.3 c.c. greater than his stated minimum value of 87.0 c.c. for a sample of 86 crania, while the higher values range right up to 40.7 c.c. greater than the mean. If correct, these figures represent so extreme a departure from the patterns of other hominoid distributions, including that of another hylobatine sample, the siamang, that it was strongly suspected a typographical or other error had crept into the data tabulated for gibbons in Vallois's paper (1954).

In a letter in response to my inquiry, M. Vallois has indeed indicated that the published mean of 89.3 c.c. was erroneous and that the mean value should be 94.3 c.c. This figure, he stated, was based on Schultz's (1933) data for 77 gibbons of both sexes, coupled with Vallois's own data for 9 gibbons of both sexes. Even the revised mean of 94.3 gives an unusually asymmetrical distribution if the minimum and maximum values have been correctly cited. However, reference to Schultz's original (1933) paper revealed that the range cited by Vallois (1954) was not correct. Schultz's (1933) data for 77 gibbons of both sexes show a range of capacities from 70 to 136 c.c., whereas Vallois's stated range for 86 gibbons (which included Schultz's 77) was 87 to 130 c.c. It is possible that the shorter range represents that of only the 9 gibbon capacities that Vallois himself added to Schultz's 77 capacities. The total range culled from Schultz (1933) is much more symmetrical than Vallois's range. If we accept Vallois's new mean for the 86 capacities, namely 94.3 c.c., then the minimum value (70 c.c.) is 24.3 c.c., or 2.2 estimated S.D.s, below the sample mean, while the maximum value (136 c.c.) is 41.7 c.c., or 3.8 S.D.s, above the sample mean. If we follow Schultz's mean of 97.5 c.c. for 77 gibbons of both sexes, the minimum capacity (70 c.c.) is 27.5 c.c., or 2.5 estimated S.D.s below the mean, while the maximum value (136 c.c.) is 38.5 c.c., or 3.5 estimated S.D.s, above the mean. This represents a positively skewed distribution, comparable with that for the gorilla combined-sex sample shown in Table 12.

A serious objection to using either Schultz's 77 or Vallois's 86 gibbon capacities in Tables 4, 9, and 12 is that their samples are made up from several different hylobatine species, whereas the figures for each of the other hominoids cited are for samples drawn from a single species. Thus, Schultz's 77 gibbon capacities comprise 28 of *Hylobates lar*, 21 of *H. agilis*, 10 of *H. cinereus*, 9 of *H. pileatus*, 6 of *H. concolor*, and 3 of *H. hoolock* (but exclude 10 of *H. klossii*).

Hence, the figures based on these 77 crania and on Vallois's 86 crania have here been discarded. To elucidate the question further, I approached Dr. A. Schultz, and he very kindly provided me with the original, unpublished raw data for the series described in his 1944 monograph. These data are the cranial capacities of 95 male and 85 female fully adult, wild

TABLE 12: *Symmetry and skewing of samples of hominoid cranial capacities*

Species and sample	Sample mean (in c.c.)	S.D. of mean (in c.c.)	Absolute value (in c.c.)	Highest observed value Deviation from mean (in c.c.)	Standardized deviation from mean (in S.D.s)
GIBBON					
(*Hylobates lar*)					
Males (*n* = 95)	104.0	7.51	125.0	+21.0	+2.79
Females (*n* = 85)	100.9	7.81	116.0	+15.1	+1.93
Combined males and females (*n* = 180)	102.5	7.81	125.0	+22.5	+2.88
GIBBON					
(*Hylobates agilis*)					
Combined males and females (*n* = 21)	98.8	10.32	120.0	+21.1	+2.05
SIAMANG					
(*Symphalangus syndactylus*)					
Males (*n* = 23)	125.8	12.95	150.0	+24.2	+1.87
Females (*n* = 17)	122.8	13.09	152.0	+29.2	+2.23
CHIMPANZEE					
(*Pan troglodytes*)					
Males (*n* = 24)	420.0	33.33	480.0	+60.0	+1.80
Males (*n* = ?)	404.3	?	470.0	+65.7	?
Males (*n* = 34)	399.5	40.61	500.0	+100.5	+2.47
Males (*n* = 56)	381.0	35.29	454.0	+73.0	+2.07
Pooled males (*n* = 163)	398.5	38.88	500.0	+101.5	+2.61
Females (*n* = 26)	390.0	32.83	450.0	+60.0	+1.83
Females (*n* = ?)	388.8	?	440.0	+51.2	?
Females (*n* = 27)	365.8	33.70	455.0	+89.2	+2.65
Females (*n* = 57)	350.0	28.85	415.0	+65.0	+2.25
Pooled females (*n* = 200)	371.1	32.42	460.0	+88.9	+2.74
Combined males and females (*n* = 144)	393.8	30.36	480.0	+86.2	+2.84
Combined males and females (*n* = 363)	383.4	37.14	500.0	+116.6	+3.14

Hylobates lar from a very limited district in northern Thailand. The data, as reduced by my research assistants, Miss C. J. Orkin, C. Block, and M. Hockman, are recorded in Tables 4, 9, and 12. Table 12 shows a slightly positively skewed distribution for male *H. lar* and a very slightly negatively skewed, or virtually symmetrical, distribution for female *H. lar*.

Of the various other subsamples of gibbons cited by Oppenheim (1911–1912) and Schultz (1933), only that of *H. agilis* is perhaps big enough to be cited in my tables. Oppenheim recorded the mean and range for 8 specimens of unknown sex, and Schultz the raw data for 8 males and

Absolute value (in c.c.)	Lowest observed value Deviation from mean (in c.c.)	Standardized deviation from mean (in S.D.s)	Algebraic sum of deviations of highest and lowest observed values Absolute value (in c.c.)	Standardized value (in S.D.s)	Comment
89.0	−15.0	−2.00	+6.0	+0.79	Slightly positively skewed
82.0	−18.9	−2.42	−3.8	−0.49	Slightly negatively skewed
82.0	−20.5	−2.62	+2.0	+0.26	± Symmetrical
81.0	−17.8	−1.72	+3.4	+0.33	± Symmetrical
100.0	−25.8	−1.99	−1.6	−0.12	± Symmetrical
105.0	−17.8	−1.36	+11.4	+0.87	Slightly positively skewed
350.0	−70.0	−2.10	−10.0	−0.30	± Symmetrical
350.0	−54.3	?	+11.4	?	± Symmetrical
325.0	−74.5	−1.83	+26.0	+0.64	Slightly positively skewed
292.0	−89.0	−2.52	−16.0	−0.45	Slightly negatively skewed
292.0	−106.5	−2.74	−5.0	−0.13	± Symmetrical
320.0	−70.0	−2.13	−10.0	−0.30	± Symmetrical
350.0	−38.8	?	+12.4	?	± Symmetrical
290.0	−75.8	−2.25	+13.4	+0.40	Slightly positively skewed
282.0	−68.0	−2.36	−3.0	−0.11	± Symmetrical
282.0	−89.1	−2.75	−0.2	−0.01	Symmetrical
320.0	−73.8	−2.43	+12.4	+0.41	Slightly positively skewed
282.0	−101.4	−2.73	+15.2	+0.41	Slightly positively skewed

5 females. The pooled data give a sample of 21 capacities for *H. agilis* of both sexes. The combined sample mean, as given by Schultz (1933), is 98.8 c.c., and the combined sample range is 81 to 120 c.c. These figures are used as a basis for a further series of *Hylobates* entries in Tables 4, 9, and 12. The distribution in *H. agilis,* as Table 12 shows, is virtually symmetrical.

It became clear that Vallois's cited data for 40 siamang (*Symphalangus syndactylus*) were those of Oppenheim (*n* = 26) together with those of Schultz (*n* = 14). From the original references (Oppenheim 1911–1912;

TABLE 12 (*Continued*)

	Sample mean (in c.c.)	S.D. of mean (in c.c.)	Highest observed value		
Species and sample			Absolute value (in c.c.)	Deviation from mean (in c.c.)	Standardized deviation from mean (in S.D.s)
ORANGUTAN (*Pongo pygmaeus*)					
Males (*n* = ca. 80)	455.0	35.05	530.0	+75.0	+2.14
Males (*n* = ?)	395.0	?	480.0	+85.0	?
Males (*n* = 36)	434.1	50.86	523.0	+88.9	+1.75
Males (*n* = 57)	416.0	36.44	502.0	+86.0	+2.36
Pooled males (*n* = 203)	434.4	39.93	540.0	+105.6	+2.64
Females (*n* = ca. 70)	390.0	39.92	490.0	+100.0	+2.51
Females (*n* = ?)	357.6	?	390.0	+32.4	?
Females (*n* = 59)	389.8	36.27	494.0	+104.2	+2.87
Females (*n* = 52)	338.0	32.89	425.0	+87.0	+2.65
Pooled females (*n* = 199)	374.5	38.65	494.0	+119.5	+3.09
Combined males and females (*n* = 260)	411.2	31.75	475.0	+63.8	+2.01
Combined males and females (*n* = 402)	404.8	44.44	540.0	+135.2	+3.04
GORILLA (*G. gorilla gorilla*)					
Males (*n* = 50)	510.0	37.78	590.0	+80.0	+2.12
Males (*n* = 22)	505.4	?	585.0	+79.6	?
Males (*n* = 26)	550.6	59.44	655.0	+104.4	+1.76
Males (*n* = 23)	513.0	50.71	652.0	+139.0	+2.74
Males (*n* = 133)	543.0	50.00	685.0	+142.0	+2.84
Males (*n* = 72)	535.0	71.13	752.0	+217.0	+3.05
Pooled males (*n* = 400)	534.8	55.89	752.0	+217.2	+3.89
Pooled males (*n* = 414)	534.6	57.05	752.0	+217.4	+3.81
Females (*n* = 48)	450.0	33.56	530.0	+80.0	+2.38
Females (*n* = 78)	461.0	47.70	580.0	+119.0	+2.49
Females (*n* = 43)	443.0	39.41	523.0	+80.0	+2.03
Pooled females (*n* = 254)	455.6	45.13	595.0	+139.4	+3.09
Combined males and females (*n* = 532)	497.8	56.46	685.0	+187.2	+3.37
Combined males and females (*n* = 653)	506.0	66.03	752.0	+246.0	+3.73
Combined males and females (*n* = 668)	504.6	65.92	752.0	+247.4	+3.75
MODERN MAN (*Homo sapiens*)					
Males (*n* = 1000s)	1345.0	200.00	2100	+755.0	+3.78
	1345.0	169.00	2000	+655.0	+3.88

	Lowest observed value		Algebraic sum of deviations of highest and lowest observed values		
Absolute value (in c.c.)	Deviation from mean (in c.c.)	Standardized deviation from mean (in S.D.s)	Absolute value (in c.c.)	Standardized value (in S.D.s)	Comment
360.0	−95.0	−2.71	−20.0	−0.57	Slightly negatively skewed
320.0	−75.0	?	+10.0	?	± Symmetrical
343.0	−91.1	−1.79	−2.2	−0.04	± Symmetrical
334.0	−82.0	−2.25	+4.0	+0.11	± Symmetrical
320.0	−114.4	−2.87	−8.8	−0.23	± Symmetrical
300.0	−90.0	−2.25	+10.0	+0.26	± Symmetrical
300.0	−57.6	?	−25.2	?	Slightly negatively skewed
304.0	−85.8	−2.37	+18.4	+0.50	Slightly positively skewed
276.0	−62.0	−1.89	+15.0	+0.76	Slightly positively skewed
276.0	−98.5	−2.55	+21.0	+0.54	Slightly positively skewed
295.0	−116.2	−3.66	−52.4	−1.65	Negatively skewed
276.0	−128.8	−2.90	+6.4	+0.14	± Symmetrical
420.0	−90.0	−2.38	−10.0	−0.26	± Symmetrical
420.0	−85.4	?	−5.8	?	± Symmetrical
450.0	−100.6	−1.69	+3.8	+0.07	± Symmetrical
440.0	−73.0	−1.44	+66.0	+1.30	Positively skewed
420.0	−123.0	−2.46	+19.0	+0.38	± Symmetrical
412.0	−123.0	−1.73	+94.0	+1.32	Positively skewed
420.0	−114.8	−2.05	+102.4	+1.84	Positively skewed
412.0	−122.6	−2.15	+94.8	+1.66	Positively skewed
380.0	−70.0	−2.09	+10.0	+0.29	± Symmetrical
340.0	−121.0	−2.54	−2.0	−0.05	± Symmetrical
350.0	−93.0	−2.36	−13.0	−0.33	± Symmetrical
340.0	−115.6	−2.56	+23.8	+0.53	Slightly positively skewed
340.0	−157.8	−2.79	+29.4	+0.58	Slightly positively skewed
340.0	−166.0	−2.51	+80.0	+1.22	Positively skewed
340.0	−164.6	−2.50	+82.8	+1.25	Positively skewed
800.0	−545.0	−2.73	+210.0	+1.05	Positively skewed
900.0	−445.0	−2.63	+210.0	+1.25	Positively skewed

Schultz 1933) it was possible to divide the combined sample of 40 into separate male and female subsamples of 23 and 17, respectively. Since such data are clearly more valuable than those for combined-sex samples, the newly computed data for male and female siamangs separately are included in Tables 4, 9, and 12. These show that the capacities for 23 male siamangs are symmetrically distributed, whereas those for the smaller sample of 17 female siamangs are slightly positively skewed.

To summarize on the hylobatines, for male and female *H. lar* the differences between the deviations of the smallest and largest values for each sample are 0.79 S.D.s and 0.49 S.D.s, respectively, while for the small samples of *H. agilis* (combined sexes) and male and female siamangs the corresponding differences are 0.33 S.D.s, 0.12 S.D.s, and 0.87 S.D.s, respectively. If we regard values of less than 0.40 as representing symmetry, values between 0.41 and 1.00 as indicating slight skewness, and values of over 1.00 as showing definite skewness, all of these hylobatine values may be considered small enough to permit the distribution curves to be regarded as virtually symmetrical or, at most, only slightly skewed.

In the chimpanzee sample the maximum and minimum values for pooled one-sex samples are close to 3 standard deviations above and below the mean, respectively (Table 12). The neglible difference between the deviations of the 2 extreme values is −0.13 S.D.s for males and −0.01 S.D.s for females.

For orangutan capacities, the male distribution curve is very slightly skewed to the left. The highest value (540 c.c.) is 2.64 S.D.s above the sample mean, whilst the lowest value (320 c.c.) is 2.87 S.D.s below the mean. The difference between the deviations of the 2 extreme values in the sample is −0.23 S.D.s. On the other hand, the female orang sample is slightly positively skewed, the difference of the extreme deviations being +0.54 S.D.s. However, these asymmetries are again slight and compare well with the values for hylobatines. The overall effect is of symmetrically distributed samples of orangutan capacities. It is interesting to note, however, that Vallois's combined-sex sample of 260 capacities is definitely negatively skewed, the highest value being only 2.01 S.D.s above the sample mean, whereas the lowest value is no less than 3.66 S.D.s below the mean. I drew attention to this apparently exceptional distribution in a previous publication (Tobias 1968b). No fewer than 2 of the orang subsamples, Selenka's males and Oppenheim's females, show slight negative skewing, 5 are more or less symmetrical, and 3 are slightly positively skewed (Table 12). However, the appreciable negative skewing that characterized Vallois's combined-sex sample of 260 capacities is not a feature of my own combined-sex pooled sample of 402 capacities. The latter distribution has maximum and minimum values almost exactly 3 S.D.s above and below the mean (as is to be expected in a normally distributed variate when $n = 442$).

The gorilla samples are strongly positively skewed in males and slightly in females. The differences between the deviations of the extreme values are $+1.66$ S.D.s for the latest series of total pooled males, $+0.53$ S.D.s for total pooled females, and $+1.25$ S.D.s for a combined-sex pooled sample.

Similarly, the modern human sample is definitely positively skewed, 2 outside estimates giving differences between the extreme deviations of $+1.05$ and $+1.25$ S.D.s.

Thus, 4 of the hominoid samples cited, namely gibbon, siamang, chimpanzee, and orangutan, have virtually symmetrical distributions; and 2, gorilla and modern man, have positively skewed distributions.

THE MEANING OF THE VARIABLE DISTRIBUTION OF CRANIAL CAPACITIES. The different kinds and degrees of skewing that the figures in Table 12 have demonstrated pose an interesting problem.

In short, the right-skewed distributions of human and gorilla values indicate that variants with large capacity are more common than variants with small capacity in the samples representing the populations. According to Simpson et al., such moderately right-skewed distributions are common in zoology and "although an adequate census has not been made, they appear to be more common than are left-skewed distributions" (Simpson, Roe, and Lewontin 1960, p. 144). Contrariwise, the left-skewed distributions of capacities for some orangutan samples, as well as for some other hominoid series, show that small variants are more common in these samples than large variants. In most gibbon, siamang, chimpanzee, and orang samples the small and large variants occur in approximately equal frequencies.

Do these differences of distribution within a series of big hominoid samples reflect real population differences? At present, I am inclined to assume the null hypothesis and to accept that the different kinds and degrees of skewing result mainly from peculiarities of sampling rather than from population differences in the pattern of distribution of the variate. The most likely peculiarity in combined-sex samples is the sex composition of the samples: for instance, the gorilla sample of 668 capacities comprises 414 males and only 254 females.

Related to this factor, we have already examined one possible characteristic of the variate itself that may play a part, namely the existence of differing degrees of *sexual dimorphism* in cranial capacity among the various hominoid taxa, such as distinguish gorilla from chimpanzee capacities. This factor, coupled with differing proportions of the 2 sexes in the various samples, may explain some part of the differences in distribution pattern among the hominoids cited. The *age distribution* of the samples is another possibly correlated variable. Although all the samples quoted here are of adults, we do not know if the cranial capacity decreases with age. We know that brain weight and volume diminish with old age (Mettler 1955), but, to the best of my knowledge, no corresponding diminution in cranial capacity has been demonstrated, as was mentioned earlier. Hence, it remains uncertain whether age distribution of the samples has contributed to the discrepancies of skewing.

In a letter to me, Dr. T. Bielicki raised the possibility that the inclusion of different *geographical variants* may be a further factor contributing to the differences among the samples. Some of the earlier workers (for example, Selenka 1898, 1899; Gaul 1933) were at pains to distinguish such variants, recognizing larger- and smaller-brained races as represented within available samples. However, it would be most difficult, if not impossible, to obtain accurate details on the geographical provenience of all the pongid data in the literature, as authors generally have not given this information.

Simpson, Roe, and Lewontin have pointed out an interesting *statistical* reason why samples of normally distributed variates should show a small positive skew:

It may be noted that the assumption on which the use of V and the study of variability in general are based involves a constant tendency for such characters to show a small positive skew. This assumption is that the dispersion is proportionate to the absolute value of the variate. If this is true as between different samples and different variates, it should be true also within a single distribution. The absolute dispersion should tend to be, or for an average of many different homologous distributions should be, greater for higher values of the variate than for lower and should increase steadily from the left-hand end of the graphic distribution through to the right-hand end. Since the values thus tend to be spread farther on the absolute scale above the mode than below it, a positive skew is involved. . . . It is probable that the slightly skewed form of curve thus determined is a better theoretical description of most zoological variates than is the normal curve. [Simpson, Roe, Lewontin 1960, pp. 145–46]

This factor might help account for the positively skewed distributions in gorilla and man, but it makes all the more interesting the problem of the lack of positively skewed distributions in the orangutan, chimpanzee, and hylobatines.

The consequences for Australopithecus

The study of all available data has confirmed what the preliminary investigation suggested, namely that, whatever the cause or causes, the available samples of hominoid cranial capacities vary *inter se* in (a) sexual dimorphism, (b) coefficient of variability, and (c) the presence, degree, and direction of skewing of their distributions. This makes it unwarranted, even illogical, to base a correction factor for a fossil group such as *Australopithecus* on one or another living hominoid. In particular, it is highly arbitrary to select the 2 positively skewed samples (man and gorilla) to derive a correction factor that would skew the distribution curve of australopithecine capacities so far to the right as to permit the estimated population range to reach 680 c.c. (the original estimate of the endocranial capacity for the type specimen of *H. habilis*), as Robinson has done (1966).

It is concluded that, on grounds of variable skewness as well as variable variability of available hominoid samples of capacities, it would be arbitrary and of doubtful validity to select one or another skewed sample of extant hominoid capacities to estimate the possible maximum value in an extinct and poorly represented fossil taxon. Certainly, estimates of maxima for *Australopithecus* derived in this way cannot be employed validly to assist in making a decision on systematic categories. For instance, it would not be valid to use information derived in this manner to show that the estimated cranial capacity of *H. habilis* must have fallen within the estimated population range of *A. africanus*. The only formally valid estimate of the population range of a fossil taxon such as *A. africanus* at present must be considered to be one that is based upon extrapolations from the parameters of the available fossil sample, rather than one that is based on inferences from the variable samples of living hominoid capacities. Hence, I reiterate that at this stage of our knowledge 370 to 618 c.c. represents the most reliable estimate of the population range for *Australopithecus africanus*.

FOUR

 ## THE CRANIAL CAPACITY OF HOMO HABILIS

Much controversy has been aroused since the publication in 1964 of a preliminary account of some new Olduvai remains that Leakey, Tobias, and Napier used as the type for a new hominid species, *Homo habilis*. ("Habilis" is a Latin word meaning "able, handy, mentally skillful, vigorous." The suitability of this word to designate a group that was probably responsible for the first systematic cultural stone tool-making will emerge later. The name was suggested to us by Professor Dart.)

It is not proposed here to enter into a detailed account of the controversy that has arisen around the taxonomic and phylogenetic position of the group of fossils allocated to this new taxon, nor into a discussion on its systematics. Such are at present largely premature, since no detailed and definitive account has yet been published of the specimens—these are to be featured prominently in a new volume of the *Olduvai Gorge* series. Much of the controversy and theorizing around the specimen is misplaced effort before the monographic treatment of the specimens is published.

What is relevant for this volume, however, is the fact that it has been claimed that the larger endocranial capacity of *H. habilis* is one of the criteria distinguishing it from the australopithecines.

The cranial capacity of the type specimen of
Homo habilis

On February 25, 1961, Dr. L. S. B. Leakey announced the discovery of the greater part of a juvenile hominid mandible, as well as parts of 2 beautifully preserved and undistorted parietal bones (Figure 14). The remains were found at a slightly lower level than Olduvai Hominid 5 (originally called *Zinjanthropus*), and so for some years, during the study of

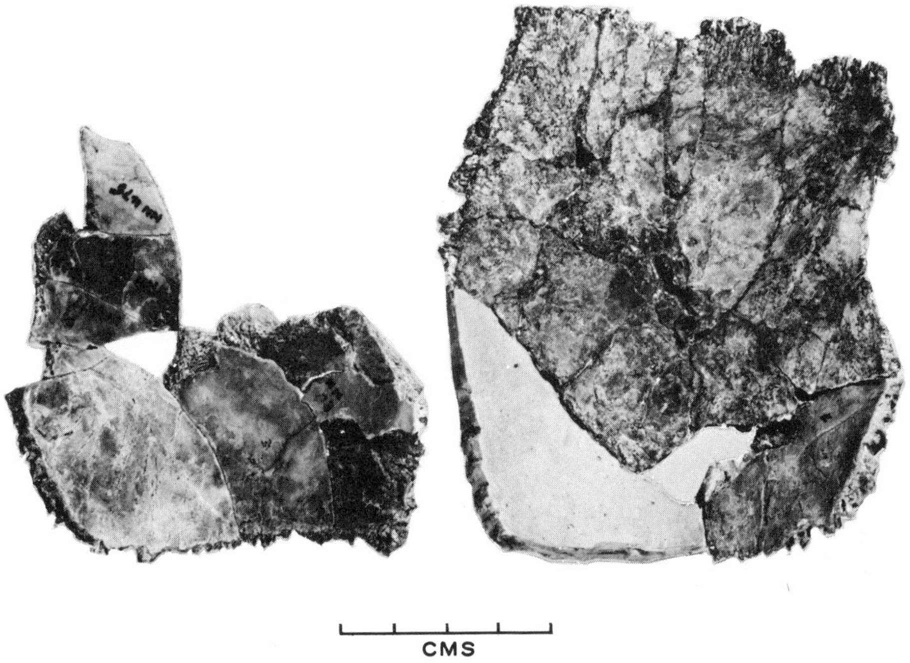

FIGURE 14: Inner aspect of the two parietal bones of the type specimen of *Homo habilis* (Olduvai hominid 7). Their measurements show that they are bigger than those of any australopithecine parietal bones yet discovered.

the new specimens, they were loosely spoken of as *pre-Zinjanthropus*. This term was used only in the sense that the type specimen came from a slightly lower level in the deposit; it was never intended that the specimen be regarded as a form ancestral to Old. Hom. 5, although some people did interpret this rather unfortunate nickname in that way. Later it was formally named *Homo habilis,* and its catalogue number is Old. Hom. 7.

Leakey (1961) pointed out that the parietals of Old. Hom. 7 were larger than those of the robust australopithecine of Olduvai; indeed they were patently larger than the parietal bones of any australopithecine yet discovered (Tobias 1966a). Thus, the sagittal arc from bregma to lambda measures 105 mm., whereas those of 5 australopithecines range from 74.5 to 91.5 mm. The squamosal arc from pterion to asterion is 69.0 mm. in *H. habilis* (type specimen) but ranges from 55.5 to 62.5 mm. in australopithecine crania. The coronal edge, although not perfectly preserved, likewise exceeds the top of the australopithecine sample range. Such large parietals necessarily covered a larger brain than that of any australopithecine known hitherto.

That fact was clearly acknowledged by Robinson in 1962, at which time he endeavored to show that early stone tools were not made by *Australopithecus* sensu stricto (i.e., *A. africanus*). In his investigation he specifically included "pre-Zinjanthropus" as a larger-brained contemporary of *A. africanus*. Thus, he stated:

In fact, there is evidence throughout the entire australopithecine period either proving or suggesting the presence of a more advanced form of hominid. There are the large parietals in the "pre-Zinj" level of Olduvai, *"Telanthropus"* at Swartkrans. . . . [Robinson 1962a, p. 102]

RECONSTRUCTING THE BIPARIETAL ARCH. It was a logical and imperative step, after the parietals had been measured, to attempt an estimate of the cranial capacity. First the missing parts of the 2 parietal bones had to be reconstructed. This was not difficult, because the entire coronal and temporal borders were present on the left bone and the entire lambdoid (or occipital) border on the right. In addition, the anterior part of the sagittal border was present on the left parietal and the posterior part of that border on the right. Further, both bones had the asterionic region intact and symmetrical.

Once the 2 bones had been thus restored, the archway formed by them had to be reconstructed (Figures 15 and 16). The first reconstruction of the biparietal part of the calvaria was made by Dr. L. S. B. Leakey and myself; later a second reconstruction was made independently by Mr. A. R. Hughes and myself. The 2 reconstructions differed from each other by a negligibly small margin: thus, the biasterionic breadth of the arch differed between the 2 reconstructions by scarcely 2 mm. (Tobias 1964, 1965a). There was possible only a narrow range of naturally appearing anatomical relationships between the left and right parietal bones: the eye soon detected the discrepancy whenever the angle between the 2 bones (along the sagittal suture) was so great or so small as to produce an appearance differing appreciably from that shown by other hominoid crania. The narrowness of this range of tolerability is testified to by the 2 mm. discrepancy between the 2 reconstructions. In any event, the irrelevance of slight and even moderate variations in this angle for the estimation of cranial capacity was effectively demonstrated by Holloway (1965), as described below.

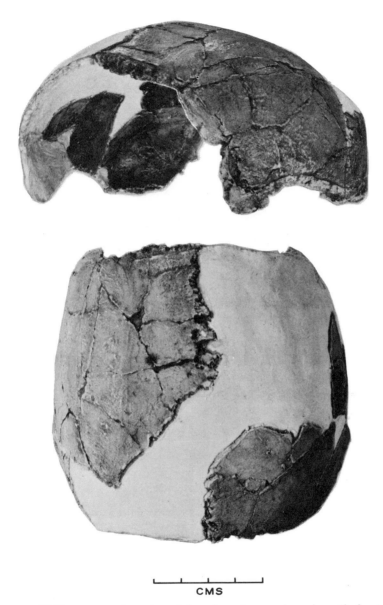

CMS

FIGURE 15: Oblique anterior view (*above*) and superior view (*below*) of the biparietal arch of Olduvai hominid 7 (the type specimen of *Homo habilis*).

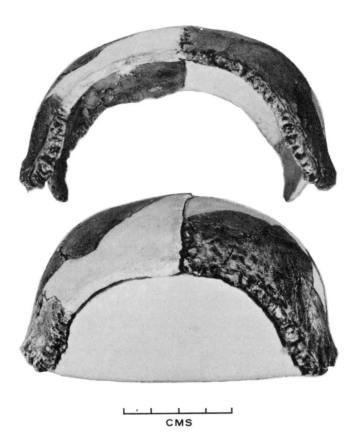

CMS

FIGURE 16: Anterior view (*above*) and posterior view (*below*) of the bi-parietal arch of Olduvai hominid 7 (the type specimen of *Homo habilis*). In the lower photograph, the artificial part-endocast is shown in position.

THE PARTIAL ENDOCAST OF OLDUVAI HOMINID 7. From the 2 reconstructed biparietal arches, partial biparietal endocasts were next made, each representing that part of the cranial cavity enclosed above and at the sides by the parietal bones (Figure 16). The front, back, and sides of the endocast were set by the borders of the articulated, reconstructed parietal bones. The basal aspect of the endocast was made to follow the concavo-convex contour of the temporal (squamosal) margins of the parietals. Each of the 2 finished products was accepted as representing the volume of the tunnel shaped space enclosed by the parietals (Figure 17).

The volume of each of the 2 partial endocasts was determined 5 times by water displacement. The endocast based on the first biparietal recon-

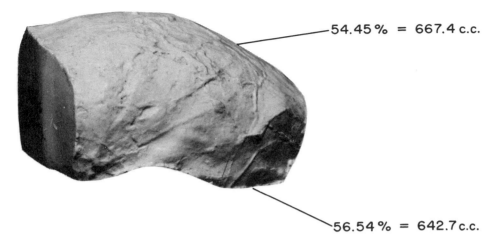

54.45% = 667.4 c.c.

56.54% = 642.7 c.c.

364 c.c.

FIGURE 17: The biparietal partial endocast of Olduvai hominid 7 (type specimen of *Homo habilis*), with outside values for the range of estimates of the total capacity. The figure of 54.45 per cent is based on *Australopithecus boisei;* that of 56.54 per cent is based on the Taung endocast of *Australopithecus africanus*. Percentages for the Trinil and Choukoutien II specimens lay between these 2 values. The central value for Olduvai hominid 7 is 657 c.c. and the estimate for the "adult value" 684 c.c.

struction yielded 5 values ranging from 362 to 364 c.c., with a mean of 363.6 c.c.; the endocast based on the second reconstruction yielded 5 values ranging from 362 to 365 c.c., with a mean of 363.4 c.c.

The validity of the method was demonstrated entirely independently by Dr. R. L. Holloway, working in the Anthropology Department of Columbia University, New York City. His work answered the criticism (voiced, for example, by Pilbeam and Simons 1965 *) that any variation in the angle between the 2 parietals would *seriously* affect the volume of the space enclosed beneath them. His experiments led him to state:

It is immediately apparent that variations in the articulation angle along the suture do not radically reduce volume estimates. In varying the articulation angle, the decrease essentially affects but one dimension, that is, the lateral breadth. At

* For example: "The slightest mis-setting of the two at the midline, for instance if flared too much laterally, would markedly increase the brain volume estimate for this individual" (Pilbeam and Simons 1965, p. 250).

65 🖋

the same time, the vertical dimension is increased . . . the loss of area from constriction of the breadth is almost compensated by the increase in depth. The [cross-sectional] area remains essentially constant, and since the length of the endocast is not affected by constriction the volume remains essentially constant also. [Holloway 1965, p. 205]

To arrive at this conclusion, Holloway varied the angle along the sagittal suture far more than necessary, that is, he increased the maximum (biasterionic) breadth by as much as 10 mm. and reduced it by as much as 20 mm. This is an extreme range, compared with the 2 mm. variation we found between our 2 reconstructions: despite his deliberate choice of what he describes as a "range surely greater than necessary," he still showed relative constancy of the volume determined. Thus, he concluded that my values for the partial endocranial volume were probably correct, provided that the reconstruction of the 2 parietal bones was valid.

CORRECTING FROM PARTIAL ENDOCAST TO THE TOTAL CRANIAL CAPACITY. And now the problem was to estimate what proportion of the total endocranial volume might be made up by the biparietal endocranial volume. In proceeding to this next step, I was simply following a long-recognized procedure in palaeoanthropology for the estimate of total from partial endocranial capacity—such, for example, as had been used by Dubois, Schaaffhausen, Schwalbe, T. H. Huxley, Sollas, and Weidenreich. What was new about this particular exercise, as far as I have been able to determine, was the use of so unusual a portion of the cranial cavity as the biparietal tunnel. Previous studies have tended to use a calotte without the calvarial base— for example Dubois's (1898) determination of the capacity of the Trinil calvaria.

To provide a basis for making my estimate, I selected 4 endocranial casts of fossil hominids in which the total volume was fairly reliably known and on which the outline of the parietal bones was unmistakeable. Two were endocasts of australopithecines (the Taung specimen and Old. Hom. 5 or *A. boisei* from Olduvai) and 2 of *Homo erectus* (1 each from Indonesia and China). From each of the 4 endocasts biparietal partial casts were prepared and the volumes determined by water displacement 5 times each. For each cast the mean values obtained were then expressed as a percentage of the known total volume.

The percentage for the Taung specimen came to 56.54; that for *A. boisei* (Old. Hom. 5) came to 54.45 (Figure 18); and that for *H. erectus pekinensis* came to 54.64 (Figure 19). The value for the Trinil specimen,

54.5 %

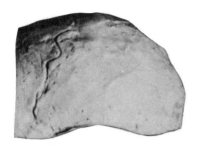
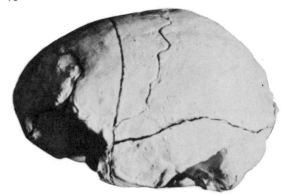

289 c.c.   **530 c.c.**

FIGURE 18: The biparietal partial endocast and the total endocast of Olduvai hominid 5 (type specimen of *Australopithecus boisei*).

based on Dubois's figure of 935 c.c., came to 50.22 per cent. Since then, I have had the opportunity of reestimating the total volume of the Trinil specimen (see chapter on *Homo erectus*, p. 81): it amounts to 854 c.c., and so the new percentage for Trinil is 55.02 (Tobias 1967a, 1968b). This new result yields a ratio of biparietal to total endocast volume that ranges from 54.45 per cent to 56.54 per cent.

When the original list of percentages was applied to *H. habilis*, estimates were obtained that ranged from 642.7 to 723.6 c.c., with central values of 673.5 and 680.8 c.c. (Tobias 1964).

When the revised list of percentages, modified by the new value for Trinil, is applied to *H. habilis*, somewhat lower values are obtained: the range of estimates now becomes 642.7 to 667.4 c.c. (Figure 17), with a central value of 657 c.c. instead of the former estimate of 675 to 680 c.c (Tobias 1968b, p. 83).

The new revised estimate of 657 c.c. for the type specimen of *H. habilis* exceeds my new estimate of the *A. africanus* mean of 494 c.c. by 163 c.c., or 3.93 S.D.s. This value is extremely high and confirms that the estimated cranial capacity of the type specimen of *H. habilis* is significantly greater than the mean capacity of the available sample of *A. africanus* capacities.

If we compare the value of 657 c.c. with Robinson's proposed new mean for *A. africanus*, namely 430 c.c., the excess is 277 c.c. or 5.47 S.D.s (by my estimate, i.e., S.D. = 41.5 c.c.) or 4.54 S.D.s (by Robinson's

67 🖋

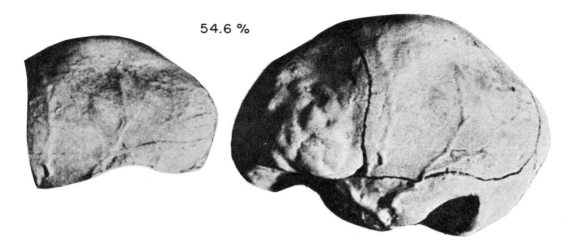

54.6 %

563 c.c.   1030 c.c.

FIGURE 19: The biparietal partial endocast and the total endocast of *Homo erectus pekinensis* II from Choukoutien, China.

estimate, i.e., S.D. = 50 c.c.). Both of these values exceed, in number of S.D.s in excess of the mean, the maximum values computed for living hominoids (see Table 7), namely +3.88 and +3.78 for man, +3.89 or +3.81 for male gorilla, and +3.75 for male and female gorilla.

In relation to my estimate of the *A. africanus* mean (494 c.c.), the *H. habilis* excess of 3.93 S.D.s just exceeds the greatest excesses in the list (those of modern man and of gorilla males) but far exceeds those of orangutan and chimpanzee, as well as the limits customarily accepted as indicating a significant difference for a normally distributed variate. Clearly, the type specimen of *H. habilis* of Olduvai was significantly larger-brained than *A. africanus* of South Africa.*

CORRECTING FOR THE JUVENILE AGE OF OLDUVAI HOMINID 7. The foregoing discussion, it must be remembered, has been based on a capacity estimated for a juvenile specimen. Should the value be corrected in order to obtain the "adult value" of *H. habilis?* The dental age of the type specimen is, by modern standards, about twelve years, the second molars

---

* Holloway's (1970) calculations likewise show a significant difference between the capacity estimated for Old. Hom. 7 (657 c.c.) and that for gracile australopithecines of South Africa. The figure of 657 c.c. exceeds by 215 c.c., or 9.96 S.D., his mean of 442 for the gracile australopithecines; if the mean of 450 c.c. is considered, the excess is 207 c.c., or 9.20 S.D.s.

having just erupted. Its individual age would have been at least three or four years younger than that of Old. Hom. 5 (*A. boisei*). Thus, whereas it was not deemed necessary to allow for a correction factor in the latter specimen, whose third molars are erupting but have not quite reached the occlusal plane, in the case of Old. Hom. 7 such a correction should perhaps be made.

Growth data on living hominoids. There is a dearth of data for other specimens of the same dental age. Selenka is quoted by Zuckerman (1928) as stating that after the eruption of the second permanent molar in the chimpanzee the capacity was 94 to 97 per cent of the adult size; unfortunately, this was apparently based on only 4 skulls. The average capacity for Zuckerman's 7 chimpanzees at the "intermediate stages" was 97.5 per cent of the adult. This intermediate stage is not, however, confined to ages after eruption of the second molars but covers all specimens between those showing "milk teeth plus first permanent molars" to the stage designated "third molar unerupted." Hence, Zuckerman's "intermediate" group may have included individuals younger than the type specimen of *H. habilis.*

Ashton and Spence (1958) used a somewhat differently defined "intermediate stage." The lower limit for their intermediate category seems to have been exactly the same as that used by Zuckerman (1928). That is, the skulls must have more permanent teeth than the first molar (and, in the case of man, possibly also more than the permanent central incisors). However, the upper limit differs: whereas Zuckerman uses a further subadult stage ("third molar unerupted"), Ashton and Spence have no further subadult stage; their ensuing stage is defined as "Adults with all permanent teeth fully erupted." Thus, while the specimens in their intermediate category, "stage c," may have included some representing individuals younger than the type specimen of *H. habilis,* the category may likewise have included some older ones, sufficiently older to have reached the probable value of 100 per cent of adult cranial capacity. For immature specimens, Ashton and Spence did not separate capacities for males and females but rather lumped them into a single combined-sex category and compared their mean with that of a combined-sex sample of adults.

The figures cited by Ashton and Spence for 4 living hominoids are as follows (I have included in parentheses 2 amendments based on my own computations from the actual means given by these workers): *

* Table after Ashton and Spence 1958, p. 171.

Species	Mean at intermediate age—"stage c" (in c.c.) (males and females)	Mean at adult age —"stage d" (in c.c.) (males and females)	Percentage
Chimpanzee	375	390	97 (96.1)
Gorilla	490	510	96
Orangutan	385	400	97 (96.25)
Man ("mixed stock")	1230	1320	93

Thus, for all 3 of the great apes, the value is 96 per cent, whilst for man it is somewhat lower, namely 93 per cent.

Schultz (1965) has used an intermediate category designated "Juvenile II," which is identical with that of Ashton and Spence; that is, it is the last subadult category. Furthermore, although the samples are of limited size, he has separated the sexes and quotes figures for each alone. His percentages are as follows: *

Species	Mean—juvenile II (in c.c.)		Mean—adult (in c.c.)		Percentage	
	males	females	males	females	males	females
Chimpanzee	370	351	381	350	97	100
Gorilla	505	431	535	443	94	97
Orangutan	380	329	416	338	91	97
Man (Black and White)	1388	—	1428	—	97	—

A summary of the data given by Ashton and Spence and by Schultz is as follows:

Species	Percentages		
	males	females	males and females
Chimpanzee	97	100	96 or 97
Gorilla	94	97	96
Orangutan	91	97	96 or 97
Man	97	—	93
Mean	95	98	95.5

From the data given by Selenka, Zuckerman, Ashton and Spence, and Schultz, it would seem likely that if ancient hominids resembled

* Table after Schultz 1965, Tables 3, 4, 5, and 6.

modern hominoids in growth pattern of the cranial cavity, a figure between 95 and 98 per cent, say 96.5 per cent, or the mean for both sexes, 95.5 per cent, would probably give a realistic assessment of the adult capacity that the type specimen of *H. habilis* had attained at the time of the individual's death. This figure may err somewhat on the conservative side, in view of the relatively low value (93 per cent) cited by Ashton and Spence for man; on the other hand, Schultz's figure for human males is higher (97 per cent). It should be recalled that the figures of 95.5 and 96.5 per cent are based upon intermediate categories, possibly including individuals both dentally younger and dentally older than the *H. habilis* type specimen.

The mean between the male and female averages for the 4 hominoids is 96.5 per cent according to Schultz, while the combined-sex mean for the same 4 hominoids is 95.5 per cent according to Ashton and Spence. The intermediate value of 96 per cent would seem to be a not unlikely estimate of the probable percentage of adult capacity attained by the type specimen of *H. habilis,* without begging the question as to its sex.

The "adult capacity" of Olduvai Hominid 7. If then we assume that at 657 c.c. the endocranial capacity of *H. habilis* was already 96 per cent of the adult value, the adult value would have been 684 c.c. We are back where we were, close to the upper part of the original 2 central estimates for *H. habilis* type (675 and 680 c.c.), only with much greater confidence in the validity of our estimate. It is proposed, therefore, that we accept the figure of 684 c.c. as the "adult value" for the type specimen of *H. habilis.*

Thus, in relation to my estimate of the mean for *A. africanus* (494 c.c.), the "adult" of *H. habilis* type shows an excess of 190 c.c., or 4.58 S.D.s. In relation to Robinson's estimate of the mean for *A. africanus* (430 c.c.), the "adult value" of *H. habilis* type shows an excess of 254 c.c. This is equivalent to an excess of 6.12 S.D.s by my estimate of the S.D. (41.5 c.c.) and of 5.08 S.D.s by Robinson's estimate of the S.D. (50 c.c.). All 3 values for standardized excesses of the *H. habilis* type "adult" capacity over the mean for *A. africanus* exceed the greatest standardized excesses tabulated in Table 12.*

* In relation to Holloway's mean of 442 c.c., the adult value of 684 c.c. is 242 c.c. in excess, which, according to an S.D. of 21.59 c.c., is equivalent to an excess of 11.21 S.D.s. In comparison with my modification of Holloway's mean (450 c.c.), the adult value for Old. Hom. 7 is 234 c.c. in excess, which, according to an S.D. of 22.49 c.c., is equivalent to an excess of 10.40 S.D.s.

The corrected adult value for the type specimen of *H. habilis* (684 c.c.) is even more significantly in excess of the *A. africanus* mean than the earlier computations showed. Furthermore, this value lies very much closer to the smallest *H. erectus* value on record (750 c.c.) than to the largest *A. africanus* capacity estimated (540 c.c.): the differences are 66 c.c. and 144 c.c., respectively!

The cranial capacity of Olduvai Hominid 13
(paratype of H. habilis)

In 1964, Dr. and Mrs. Leakey reported the discovery in October 1963 of many parts of a small skull at the site MNK II, Olduvai Gorge. The fragments came from a level some 25 feet above the marker tuff, *If,* at the base of Bed II. They comprised the vault associated with the greater part of a mandible and parts of both maxillae, all the mandibular teeth and some of the maxillary cheek teeth, The lower third molars were fully erupted, but as yet unworn, and the upper third molars were just emerging from the alveoli. A dental age intermediate between that of Old. Hom. 7 (the type specimen of *H. habilis*) and that of Old Hom. 5 (the type specimen of *A. boisei*) is indicated, that is, late adolescence. The specimen has been recorded as Old. Hom. 13, and it has been assigned as a paratype of *H. habilis* (Leakey, Tobias, and Napier 1964).

Aside from the preliminary description in 1964, the jaws and teeth have been subjected to a preliminary study, and resemblances between them and certain of the Javanese remains (Sangiran B mandible and the maxilla of *"Pithecanthropus IV"*) have been pointed out (Tobias and von Koenigswald 1964). We stressed, however (ibid., p. 516), that these resemblances applied only to the teeth and jaws. We by no means intended to convey the impression that the total creature, represented by Old. Hom. 13, was close in morphology to *H. erectus:* to do so would have been premature at that stage when we were still working on the reconstruction of the cranium. In 1966 I clarified this point further, as follows:

Whether the Bed II hominine *as a whole* parallels the Javanese *H. erectus* remains to be seen when the rest of the cranium has been studied. Until such time, Hominid 13 remains as a paratype of *H. habilis,* in accordance with the rules of zoological nomenclature. No formal proposal has yet been made to remove it from the paratypes of *H. habilis.* [Tobias 1966b, p. 579]

Unfortunately, some workers have rather prematurely come to regard the entire specimen Old. Hom. 13 as *Homo erectus* (e.g., Bielicki 1966;

Robinson 1965), but this is by no means supported by the evidence. Some of this evidence I am presenting here for the first time.

In 1966 I effected a reconstruction of most of the posterior two-thirds of the vault of the cranium (Figure 20). The reconstruction includes the 2 parietals and the occipital (as far forward as the posterior intra-occipital synchondrosis, which has, of course, long since ossified). Parts of the frontal and of the right temporal bones articulate with the rest, but for purposes of computing the endocranial volume they have been omitted from the reconstruction. Thus, the proportion of vault available for the making of a partial endocast is greater than was the case with the type specimen of *H. habilis* (where no occipital was included).

Within the incomplete reconstructed vault, R. J. Clarke made a partial endocranial cast. Anteriorly, this was smoothed off flush with the plane of what I recorded in my notes as "an apparent portion of the coronal suture." Inferiorly, the notch in the squamosal margin of the parietal was carried right across the basal surface of the endocast, as was done in the making of the part-endocast of Old. Hom. 7. Postero-inferiorly, the plane of truncation of the endocast passed just behind the foramen magnum and traversed the impression of the cerebellar hemisphere on each side. The endocast thus included all that part of the endocranial cavity cut off beneath the biparietal tunnel, together with that portion continued within the concavity of the squama occipitalis.

Comparable truncated part-casts were made of the endocasts of Old. Hom. 5 (*A. boisei*) and of Sts 5 (*A. africanus*). The casts were then varnished with shellac and their volumes determined by volumetric displacement of water, 6 times each.

The 6 estimates of the part-cast of Old. Hom. 13 yielded values of 389, 389, 391, 393, 394, and 394 c.c. The mean of the 6 readings was 391.67 c.c. The 6 readings for Sts 5 ranged from 292 to 295 c.c. and gave a mean value of 293.67 c.c. This amounted to 61.2 per cent of the estimated total of 480 c.c. (or 60.6 per cent of Holloway's estimated total of 485 c.c.). The 6 readings for Old. Hom. 5 ranged from 322 to 328 c.c., with a mean of 325.5 c.c. This amounted to 61.4 per cent of the estimated total of 530 c.c.

Thus, the 2 specimens used as analogues yielded ratios of 61.2 (or 60.6) and 61.4 per cent. When the value for the part-endocast of Old. Hom. 13 is brought up to 100 per cent on this basis, capacities of 640.0 and 637.9 c.c. are obtained, or, in round figures, 638 to 640 c.c. The midvalue of the 2 estimates is 639 c.c. Thus, the estimate for the paratype of *H. habilis* is only

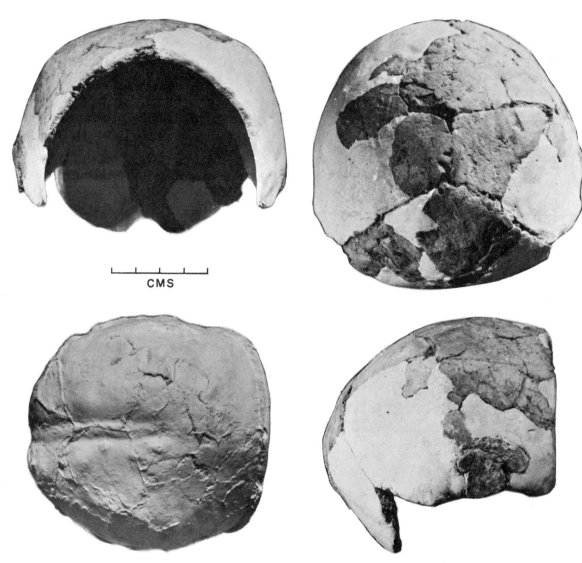

CMS

FIGURE 20: Three views of part of the reconstructed vault of the cranium of Olduvai hominid 13 (paratype of *Homo habilis*), and the artificial parieto-occipital partial endocast made by R. J. Clarke. Additional, articulating fragments of the calvaria are available but, because of their irregularity of outline, were not employed in the exercise to estimate the capacity of the calvaria.

18 c.c. less than the juvenile estimate for the type specimen (657 c.c.) and 38 c.c. less than the "adult value" for the type. On Holloway's estimate of 485 c.c. for Sts 5, a value of 646.3 c.c. is obtained for Old. Hom. 13.

Should we make an age correction for this specimen? Its dental age places it between Old. Hom. 7 (type of *H. habilis*) and Old. Hom. 5 (type of *A. boisei*). For the former we have already used a correction factor, the value being adjudged to be 96 per cent of the total; for the latter we have used no correction, the value probably being 100 per cent of the adult value. Old. Hom. 13 would seem to have been a year or two younger than *A. boisei*; it is probable that her present value would be about 98 per cent of the adult value. In this event, her "adult value" should be elevated to 652 c.c. This is 158 c.c., or 3.81 S.D.s, above my mean (494 c.c.) for *A. africanus*, and 210 c.c., or 9.73 S.D.s, above Holloway's (1970) mean of 442 c.c. On Holloway's estimate of 485 c.c. for Sts 5, Old. Hom. 13 would have an "adult value" of 660 c.c.

The cranial capacity of Olduvai Hominid 16 provisionally referred to H. habilis

In 1964 Dr. and Mrs. Leakey reported the discovery in 1963 of considerable parts of the cranial vault, as well as most of the teeth, of a young adult, "in which the third upper and lower molars are just coming into occlusion." This specimen "had been washed out by heavy rainfall at site FLK II, Maiko Gully; it had, moreover, been afterwards trampled on and very badly broken up by herds of Masai cattle before it was discovered by one of our senior African staff" (Leakey and Leakey 1964, p. 6). It was a reasonable inference that it was derived from deposits 3 to 4 feet above the marker tuff, *I¹*, at the base of Bed II, an inference since confirmed by the finding *in situ* of several teeth of the same specimen (M. D. Leakey, personal communication).

The specimen became Old. Hom. 16 in the official list of Olduvai hominids. Leakey, Tobias, and Napier (1964) did not include this specimen among the official list of paratypes of *H. habilis;* rather, it was provisionally referred to *H. habilis*. Since then a diversity of views has been expressed on this specimen by Tobias (1965b), Howell (1965), and Leakey (1966); but the full description has not yet been made. Meantime, between August 1968 and January 1969, 5 more teeth of the same individual were recovered, some *in situ*, thus virtually completing the entire set.

The new third molar is particularly instructive: it shows that not only is the crown totally unworn but the roots are not in an advanced state of formation, being very much more incomplete than in *A. boisei* (Old. Hom. 5). Thus, on dental grounds, Old. Hom. 16 is of younger individual age than Old. Hom. 5 and should perhaps be equated in age with the *H. habilis* paratype, Old. Hom. 13.

The calvaria has been reconstructed from no fewer than 107 fragments. The first reconstruction by Dr. M. D. Leakey and a modified version of it made by L. Distiller and myself on casts of the fragments were both incorrect in that an elongate fragment of bone had been placed in the left temporal fossa. As this fragment was orientated with its long axis (52.5 mm. in length) anteroposterior, it had the effect of greatly elongating the reconstructed cranium. At this stage, the reconstructed cranium had an estimated maximum glabello-occipital length of 159 to 160 mm. Furthermore, the long, ovoid appearance of the vault, as seen in norma verticalis, was strongly reminiscent of some of the Asian specimens of *H. erectus* (cf. Leakey 1966).

In January 1965, when I had the opportunity of reexamining the original fragments in Nairobi, I noticed a clear, beveled sutural edge on the

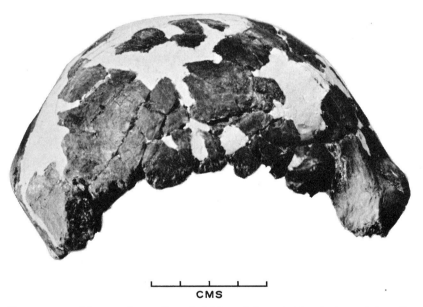

CMS

FIGURE 21: Norma lateralis of Olduvai hominid 16 (provisionally referred to *Homo habilis* by Leakey, Tobias, and Napier). The estimated cranial capacity is 620 c.c., corresponding to an "adult value" of 633 c.c.

❧ 76

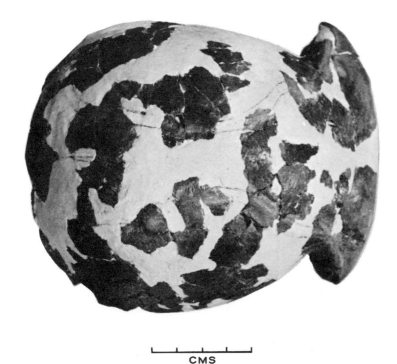

CMS

FIGURE 22: Norma verticalis of Olduvai hominid 16. This badly smashed
calvaria has been reconstructed from 107 fragments. The temporal crests
have been indicated; they do not reach the middle line.

elongate fragment, which betrayed its true identity, namely part of the right
temporal bone. The removal of the offending fragment permitted a better
alignment to be effected between the left frontal and left parietal parts (Figure 21): this converted the whole vault into a short ovoid, or even spheroid,
vault, as seen in norma verticalis (Figure 22). It resulted, too, in a maximum
glabello-occipital length of only 144 mm., that is, 15 to 16 mm. shorter than
the earlier reconstructions. The general "pithecanthropine" resemblance,
suggested by the first reconstructions—and which had led Leakey (1966) to
speak of it as "protopithecanthropine"—likewise largely disappeared.

The final reconstruction incorporates 29 fragments of the frontal, 25 of
the left parietal, 42 of the right parietal, and 11 of the occipital.

The reconstructed vault was smoothed off inferiorly with plasticine,
along a curved line corresponding closely to the lower margins of the parietals and passing through the cerebellar fossae at about the level of the posterior intra-occipital synchondrosis. The transverse limb of the cruciate

77 🖎

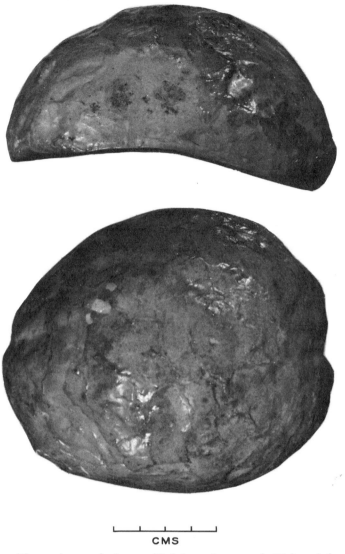

FIGURE 23: Two views of the artificial endocast of Olduvai hominid 16, made by Mr. R. J. Clarke from my reconstruction of the calvaria. The volume of the partial endocast is 410.6 c.c.; the estimated volume of the entire endocast of this adolescent is 620 c.c.

eminence was partly intact and could be reconstructed in the defective area. Thus, the lower margin of the cerebral fossae of the occipital is clear. Anteriorly, the endocranial aspect of the frontal squame is present as far as the front edge of the floor of the anterior cranial fossa.

An endocranial cast was then made by R. J. Clarke, and the base of this was smoothed and hollowed to coincide on each side with the notched lower margin of the parietal bones (Figure 23). The resulting endocast comprises a cast of the part of the braincase occupied by the major part of the cerebrum, down to the line of recurvation of the frontal lobes anteriorly and the lower margin of the occipital pole posteriorly. The parts missing comprise the cast of the rostrum, the temporal lobes, the cerebellum, and of the area occupied by the brainstem from about the level of hypothalamus to the medulla oblongata, parts that collectively seem to occupy about one-third of the total endocranial volume.

The author, assisted by Mr. Clarke, varnished the part-cast with shellac and determined its capacity by volumetric displacement of water. Eight determinations were made, and results were as follows: 408, 409, 410, 410, 411, 411, 412, and 414 c.c. The mean of the 8 readings is 410.6 c.c.

Once more, very similar part-casts were made from the 2 very complete australopithecine endocasts, namely those of Sts 5 and of Old. Hom. 5, for both of which the total endocranial volume is known (480 c.c. and 530 c.c., respectively). The part-casts were made by Mr. Clarke under the author's direction, the basal parts being removed along a curved line corresponding to the lower margin of the frontal lobe impression in front and of the occipital lobe impression behind. The volumes of the 2 part-casts were determined by 8 volumetric displacements each.

The 8 readings for Sts 5 were 317, 317, 317, 318, 319, 320, 321, and 321 c.c., giving a mean of 318.75 c.c. This value comprised 66.41 per cent of the total volume of 480 c.c. (and 65.72 per cent of Holloway's estimate of 485 c.c.). The 8 readings of Old. Hom. 5 were 345, 349, 350, 351, 352, 352, 353, and 353 c.c., giving a mean of 350.625 c.c. This value comprised 66.16 per cent of the estimated total volume of 530 c.c.

Thus, the 2 readings for the selected part-endocasts were extremely close, namely 66.41 (or 65.72) and 66.16 per cent of the respective total volumes. The total values obtained for Old. Hom. 16 on the basis of these figures amounted to 618.3 c.c. and 620.6 c.c., respectively. Using the mid-value between the 2 percentages, we obtained a value of 619.45 c.c. For practical purposes, a value of 620 c.c. may be accepted. On Holloway's estimate of 485 c.c. for Sts 5, the value for Old. Hom. 16 would be 624 c.c.

Like the previous specimen, this one represents an immature individual, and its cranial capacity may be expected to be about 98 per cent of the "adult value," as in Old. Hom. 13 (which is dentally of about the same age). If 620 c.c. represents 98 per cent of the "adult value," the total that should be recorded as the "adult value" is 633 c.c. (or, following Holloway, 638 c.c.). This value of 633 c.c. exceeds by 93 c.c. the largest estimate for an adult australopithecine of the present sample, namely 540 c.c. for the Taung "adult value." It exceeds my estimate of the mean for *A. africanus* (494 c.c.) by 139 c.c., or 3.35 S.D.s, while it surpasses Holloway's (1970) mean of 442 c.c. by 191 c.c., or 8.85 S.D.s.

Other East African hominids with habiline cranial capacities

Olduvai hominid 24, which was found in 1968 at the site DK in Bed I, possessed a severely crushed cranium and smallish teeth. It has been skillfully reconstructed by Mr. R. J. Clarke, and he has made a plaster and a plastic cast of the specimen. Mr. Clarke has kindly permitted me to quote his very tentative determination of the volume of the endocast: it is of the order of 600 c.c. but, because of crushing and distortion, may have been "well above that." Here, then, we have a fourth member of the "over 600" club from Olduvai.

Crania that may have capacities in this range—that is, about half as big again as *A. africanus*—have come to light, as well, in central and northern Kenya. At the time of writing, however, details are not available.

Summary on the cranial capacities of Olduvai Hominids 7, 13, and 16

All 3 of the Olduvai specimens that have been officially allocated or provisionally referred to *H. habilis* have capacities in the 600s, and all 3 exceed the mean for *A. africanus* from South Africa by more than 3 standard deviations. Details are as follows:

Type specimen of *H. habilis* (Old. Hom. 7)	684 c.c.
Paratype of *H. habilis* (Old. Hom. 13)	652 c.c.
Provisionally referred to *H. habilis* (Old. Hom. 16)	633 c.c.

The mean for the type and paratype of *H. habilis* comes to 668 c.c., which is 174 c.c., or 4.19 S.D.s, greater than the mean for *A. africanus* (494 c.c.). If we include the provisionally referred specimen Old. Hom. 16, the range for the 3 specimens is 633 to 684 c.c., and the mean is 656 c.c.

This value exceeds my estimated mean for *A. africanus* by 162 c.c., or 3.90 S.D.s.

Whether or not we include Old. Hom. 16 in the *H. habilis* hypodigm, it seems clear from these figures—and from the provisional estimate for Old. Hom. 24—that there existed at Olduvai some hominids possessed of significantly larger cranial capacities and, therefore, presumably of larger brains than the South African populations of *A. africanus*. This fact has been affirmed most recently by Pilbeam (1969). It assumes additional import if the Olduvai estimated capacities are compared not with my mean for *A. africanus* (494 c.c.), based on published data, but with Robinson's (1966) proposed new mean for *A. africanus* (430 c.c.), based presumably on new estimates and determinations for a sample of 6 specimens of *A. africanus.**

THE CRANIAL CAPACITY OF HOMO ERECTUS

For some time there has been a need for the redetermination of the endocranial capacities of those crania assigned to *Homo erectus*. The real want of a reassessment of the capacities of the various *H. erectus* crania became apparent to me when I had the opportunity of examining the original Indonesian material through the courtesy of Dr. D. Hooijer and Professor G. H. R. von Koenigswald. This necessity was expressed by Tobias and von Koenigswald (1964, p. 516) thus: ". . . we both feel that the capacity of the various pithecanthropine crania should be re-determined, since reconstruction of missing parts of the calvariae can now be based on better samples of related crania." In my contribution to the Juan Comas 65th Birthday Festschrift, I returned to this theme (Tobias 1965c).

Since then, the opportunity has been provided me to reassess the capacity of one of the Javanese specimens, namely Dubois's original Trinil cranium, whilst von Koenigswald has himself redetermined the capacity of another specimen. The ensuing discussion incorporates the results of these latest developments, as well as several new determinations on recently discovered specimens.

---

* Similarly with Holloway's mean of 442 c.c.

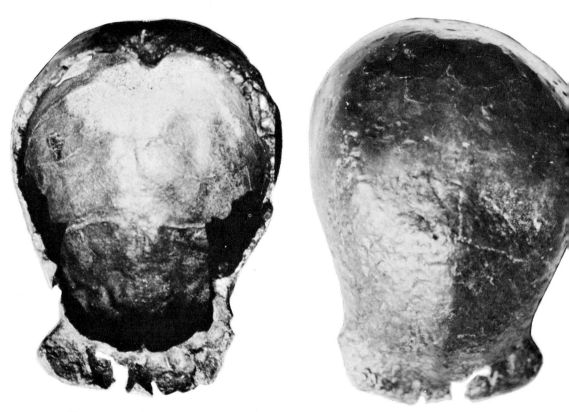

FIGURE 24: Outer and inner views of the calotte of *Homo erectus* I from Trinil, Indonesia. The capacity of the calvaria, long regarded as 900, 935, or even 950 c.c., has been redetermined as 850 c.c.

Homo erectus I of Trinil, Indonesia

The original discovery of a hominid in Java late in the last century was made by E. Dubois. The first skull was represented by little more than the calotte, or roof, of the braincase, but sufficient of the side walls of the vault and of the occipital squamous portion were preserved to enable Dubois to determine the capacity (Figure 24). It has been overlooked hitherto that, at a meeting of the Royal Dublin Society on 20 November 1895, Dubois estimated the internal capacity of the cranium as 1000 c.c. (Dubois 1895): it is clear that this was little more than a guess. In 1898 he reported to the Fourth International Congress of Zoology at Cambridge that the volume of water that could be held in the preserved part of the calvaria was 570 c.c. In order to determine what the total volume would have been, Dubois filled a number of hominoid and cercopithecoid crania up to the same level and determined the ratio between the total volume for each specimen and this part-volume (1898, 1921). The following is a list of his ratios (total/partial volumes):

Gorilla male	1.61:1	*Macaca irus* male	1.60:1
Pan troglodytes female	1.43:1	Man ("Dutch 1")	1.42:1
Pongo pygmaeus female	1.58:1	Man ("Dutch 2")	1.43:1
Hylobates agilis male	1.56:1	Man ("Dutch 3")	1.40:1
Symphalangus male	2.06:1	Man (Javanese)	1.35:1
Presbytis entellus male	1.61:1	Man (mean of 4 readings)	1.40:1

Dubois thus demonstrated that modern man differed substantially from cercopithecoids and pongids in the relative degrees of development of the upper and the lower parts of the calvaria. In modern man a larger proportion of the endocranial capacity lies *above* the plane of the maximum endocranial length. Because of the platycephaly of the Trinil calvaria, Dubois chose to compute the total volume by using the cercopithecoid and pongid ratios rather than the modern human ratio. Thus, influenced strongly by the gibbonoid aspect of the Trinil specimen's outline, he obtained a value of about 900 c.c., which he adhered to in his later discussions of the specimen (e.g., Dubois 1921, 1922, 1933). Weinert's (1928) estimate was 935 c.c. It is not quite clear whether Weidenreich (1943) accepted 935 c.c., which he quotes in the table on his p. 108, or 900 c.c., to which he refers in his text on pages 114 and 116, as discussed by Tobias (1965c, p. 382). Sartono (1968) employs Weinert's figure of 935 c.c. in his comparisons with "Pithecanthropus VII."

New estimate of cranial capacity of *Homo erectus* I. With later discoveries of more complete crania of *H. erectus* the opportunity presented itself to reassess the value for the Trinil cranium—for the astonishing fact must be recorded that most writers have gone on repeating Dubois's original (1898) estimate of 900 c.c., apparently without ever realizing that it had been based on comparison with a gibbon!

Accordingly, on 17 August 1966, with the kind help of Dr. J. T. Wiebes, Deputy Director of the Rijksmuseum voor Natuurlijke Historie, Leiden, I redetermined the part-capacity of the original Trinil specimen. Slight defects in the margin of the calotte at about the level of the maximum endocranial length were filled up with plasticine, and 3 determinations of the water content were made. These amounted to 556, 593, and 581 c.c., giving a mean of 576.67 c.c. This figure was close to the original figure of 570 c.c. cited by Dubois in 1898.

To obtain comparative data for computing the total capacity, I proceeded to Utrecht, and a week after the first determinations on the Trinil specimen, with the consent of Professor G. H. R. von Koenigswald and the help of his assistant, Miss H. Cardinaals, I determined the part-capacity of the Sangiran specimen known as *H. erectus* II of Java (Figures 25, 26, and 27). With the Sangiran calvaria filled to the same level as in the Trinil cal-

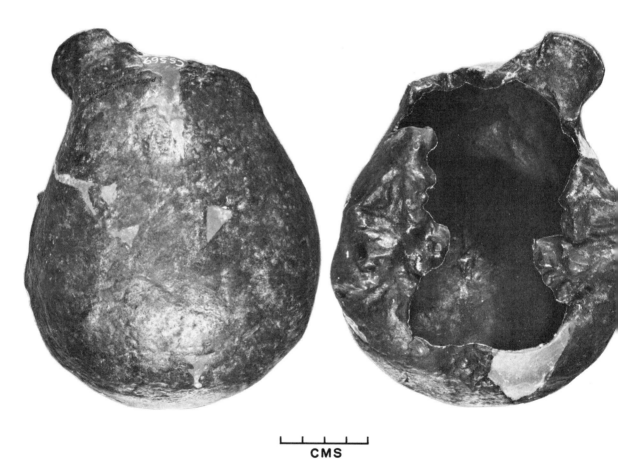

CMS

FIGURE 25: Outer and inner views of the calvaria of *Homo erectus* II from Sangiran, Indonesia. The estimated total capacity of the endocranium is 775 c.c.

❧ 84

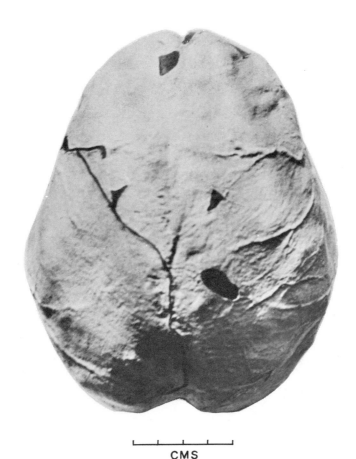

CMS

FIGURE 26: Artificial endocranial cast
of *Homo erectus* II from Sangiran, Indonesia.

varia, 3 readings of the part-capacity amounted to 516, 524, and 531 c.c., giving a mean of 523.67 c.c., or 524 c.c. to the nearest whole number. The accepted value for the total endocranial volume of Sangiran cranium II is 775
c.c. (Weidenreich 1943, pp. 115–16).* Hence, the ratio of the total volume
(775) to the part-volume (524) is 1.48:1.

When this correction factor is applied to Dubois's original part-capacity
of 570 c.c. for the Trinil calvaria, a total of 843.6 c.c. is obtained. When the

* It may be noted here that the 745 c.c. mentioned in line 5, page 115, of Weidenreich (1943) is
probably a misprint for 775 c.c., since this figure is said to be "a little more than von Koenigswald's first estimate" (which was 750 c.c.); furthermore, 775 c.c. is cited in the table on Weidenreich's page 108.

85 🖋

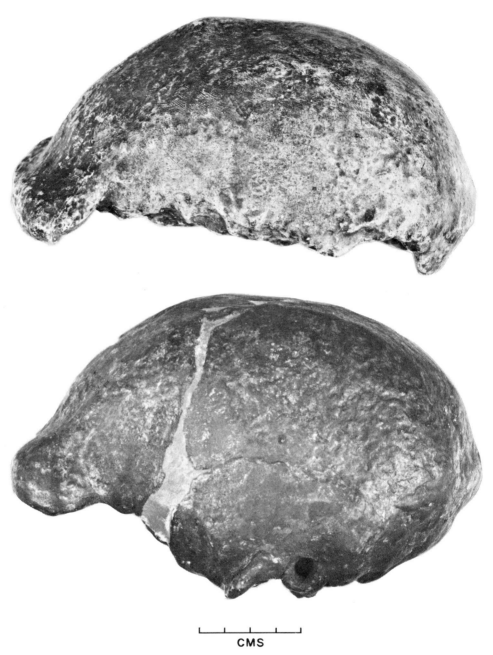

CMS

Figure 27: Norma lateralis of the calvariae of *Homo erectus* I from Trinil (*above*) and *Homo erectus* II from Sangiran (*below*). Data for the relatively complete Sangiran specimen were used by me to recompute the total capacity of the Trinil specimen.

same correction factor (1.48) is applied to my own determination of the capacity of the Trinil calvaria, a capacity of 853.5 c.c. is obtained. Thus, if *H. erectus* II had a capacity of 775 c.c., *H. erectus* I would have had a capacity of about 844 to 854 c.c., or, in round figures, 850 c.c. (Tobias 1967a). It therefore would be more correct to use the value of 850 c.c. in the future as the capacity of *H. erectus* I of Java, instead of 900 c.c. (Dubois 1898), 935 c.c. (Weinert 1928), or 900 to 950 c.c. (Äriens Kappers and Bouman 1939).

Homo erectus crania from Sangiran, Indonesia

Five crania from Sangiran have permitted estimates to be made of their internal capacity.

Homo erectus II OF INDONESIA (FIGURES 25 AND 26). This was originally estimated by von Koenigswald as having an endocranial capacity of 750 c.c. An earlier estimate by Weidenreich, subsequently disavowed by him, gave 850 c.c, while Boule and Vallois (1957) cited 815 c.c. Most workers have accepted Weidenreich's final estimate of 775 c.c. (Weidenreich 1943; Jacob 1966; von Koenigswald 1968), and this is the value I have listed in my tables (1965c, 1967a) and used for estimating the endocranial capacity of the Trinil calvaria.

Homo erectus III OF INDONESIA. This is cited by Weidenreich (1943) as having a capacity of ca. 880 c.c. and "close to 900 c.c." Both values are included in my tables, and the middle value of 890 c.c. has been used in the computation of means.

Homo erectus IV OF INDONESIA. Several years ago Dr. Wandel, under the direction of Professor von Koenigswald, completed a new reconstruction of the cranium of *H. erectus* IV, formerly ascribed by von Koenigswald to *Pithecanthropus modjokertensis* and by Weidenreich to *P. robustus*. Although his results had not yet been published, Professor von Koenigswald generously allowed me to cite the capacity he determined on Wandel's new reconstruction: it is 750 c.c. (Tobias 1967a). The new estimate of the endocranial capacity has since been published by von Koenigswald (1967).

Homo erectus VI OF INDONESIA. This cranium was discovered by a farmer in the Sangiran dome area in August 1963 (Sartono 1964; Jacob

1964, 1966). Originally it was known as "Pithecanthropus V," and as such it was listed by me (Tobias 1967a, p. 94). As explained by von Koenigswald (1968) in an appendix to the recent paper by Sartono (1968), Teuku Jacob decided subsequently to add the Modjokerto child cranium to the numbered series, and it became "Pithecanthropus V." This made the 1963 cranium "Pithecanthropus VI," or, as listed here, *H. erectus* VI. According to a letter I received from Professor von Koenigswald in 1966, the capacity is about 975 c.c. This figure was cited by Jacob (1966), while von Koenigswald (1967, p. 650) said it had a capacity of "etwa 975 cm.³" It should be reiterated that this value, entered in my list here as the capacity of *H. erectus* VI, refers to the same item as the 975 c.c. entered in my (1967a) list as that of *H. erectus* V.

Homo erectus VII of Indonesia. This cranium was found in January 1965 in the Sangiran area, though outside the actual Sangiran dome (Suradi 1965; Sartono 1967, 1968). In his 1968 paper, Sartono lists the cranial capacity as ca. 900 c.c., while in a letter to me dated 29 April 1969 Professor von Koenigswald indicated that a new reconstruction of the "Pithecanthropus VII" cranium had yielded a slightly higher capacity, namely about 930 c.c. The capacity of this cranium was not included in the up-to-date list published in the appendix to Chapter VIII of Tobias 1967a. In the present list, both values are indicated, but for purposes of calculation an intermediate value of 915 c.c. has been employed (Figure 28).

Summary on Indonesian Homo erectus

The capacities of 6 Javanese crania, 1 from Trinil and 5 from Sangiran, thus range from 750 c.c. to 975 c.c. (Table 13). Von Koenigswald's new value of 750 c.c. for *H. erectus* IV is the smallest value so far obtained for a cranium that conforms to the anatomical hallmarks of *H. erectus*. It is interesting to note that this value is just exceeded by the capacity of a single gorilla (752 c.c.—Schultz 1962).

The mean for the 6 cranial capacities is 859 c.c. The standard deviation may be computed from the size of the extreme range, with the aid of Table 6 of Lindley and Miller (1953, p. 7) and of Table 1A of Simpson, Roe, and Lewontin (1960, p. 141): it is 89 c.c. If the 6 available crania from Indonesia represent the middle reaches of the distribution for the Java-

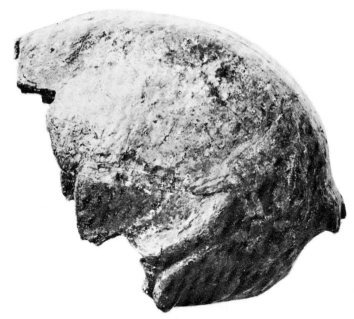

FIGURE 28: Side view of calvaria of *Homo erectus* VII from Sangiran, Indonesia. This is one of the most recently discovered *Homo erectus* crania from Indonesia and has an estimated total cranial capacity of about 915 c.c.

nese *H. erectus,* the population limits would thus be set at 592 to 1126 c.c., on the basis of 3 S.D.s above and below the sample mean.*

My Indonesian *H. erectus* series differs from that compiled by Ashton (1950). He included the 6 Ngandong crania under *"Pithecanthropus pekinensis,"* of which he states that Weidenreich (1943) gave the capacities of 11 specimens. In fact, Weidenreich gave the capacities of only 5 specimens of *P. pekinensis* (i.e., *H. erectus pekinensis*), although he mentioned another 2 estimates, 850 and 1300 c.c., in the text. When to these 5 Pekin cranial capacities are added Weidenreich's figures for the 6 Ngandong crania

* Since this passage was written, yet another cranium has come to light in the Sangiran area, namely that of *H. erectus* VIII; it was discovered on 13 September 1969 (Suradi 1969, Sartono 1970, 1971). Professor S. Sartono has very kindly permitted me to quote his unpublished estimate of the cranial capacity: it is ca. 1029 c.c. (letter from Sartono dated 30 March 1971). This is the largest capacity yet found among the 7 Indonesian crania of *H. erectus.* The range of capacities thus becomes 750 c.c. to 1029 c.c. and the new mean 883 c.c. (in place of 859 c.c.). The amended standard deviation is now estimated to be 103 c.c. instead of 89 c.c. On this basis, the population limits are widened somewhat, being set at 574 to 1192 c.c., in place of 592 to 1126 c.c.

TABLE 13: *The cranial capacity of Homo erectus* [a]

Site	Specimen	Capacity (in c.c.)	Reference
INDONESIA			
Trinil	*H. erectus erectus* I	850	Tobias 1967a
Sangiran	*H. erectus erectus* II	775	Weidenreich 1943
Sangiran	*H. erectus erectus* III	890	After Weidenreich 1943
Sangiran	*H. erectus erectus* IV	750	von Koenigswald 1967
Sangiran	*H. erectus erectus* VI	975	Jacob 1966; von Koenigswald 1967
Sangiran	*H. erectus erectus* VII	915	After Sartono 1968 and von Koenigswald, personal communication
	H. erectus erectus ($n = 6$) sample mean	859	This study
CHINA			
Choukoutien	*H. erectus pekinensis* II	1030	Weidenreich 1943
Choukoutien	*H. erectus pekinensis* III	915	Weidenreich 1943
Choukoutien	*H. erectus pekinensis* X	1225	Weidenreich 1943
Choukoutien	*H. erectus pekinensis* XI	1015	Weidenreich 1943
Choukoutien	*H. erectus pekinensis* XXI	1030	Weidenreich 1943
	H. erectus pekinensis ($n = 5$) sample mean	1043	This study
Lantian	*H. erectus* subsp.	780	Woo 1965
TANZANIA			
Olduvai	*H. erectus* subsp. (Olduvai hominid 9)	1000	Tobias 1965b
	H. erectus of Asia ($n = 12$)	929	This study
	Total *H. erectus* ($n = 13$)	935	This study

[a] Data for *H. erectus* VIII are not included in the Table (see footnotes pp. 89 and 93).

and 3 Javanese *H. erectus* crania, Ashton's total of 14 crania and his mean of 1026 c.c. are obtained. Clearly Ashton has included the 6 Ngandong crania (Ashton 1950, p. 715), although Weidenreich (1943, p. 232) indicated that he regarded them as "intermediate between the *Pithecanthropus* and *Sinanthropus* stage, on the one hand, and Neanderthal types on the other" and, again, spoke of them as representing "the next evolutionary step in the line leading from *Pithecanthropus* to modern man." The usual difficulty obtains here that intermediate or transitional forms often cannot be classified into one or another taxon under the International Code of Zoological Nomenclature (Tobias 1967b, 1969a). While Weidenreich's view would have been that Ngandong man ought to be classified as *P. soloensis*—or, by modern views, *H. erectus soloensis*—it is possible to agree with Boule and Vallois that "Ngandong man has moved sufficiently far away from *Pithecanthropus* to be regarded as a different type"; they believed then that he might be placed "in the great species of *Homo neanderthalensis,* of which he represents simply a special race" (Boule and Vallois 1957, p. 401). Since then, however, most students have ceased to regard Neandertal man as a separate species; he is commonly classified today as a subspecies of *H. sapiens.* Similarly, Campbell (1962, 1963) places Ngandong man in *H. sapiens soloensis.* Since there is certainly no agreement with Ashton (1950) that the Ngandong crania belong to *H. erectus,* I have excluded them from my *H. erectus* list (1967a).

Homo erectus from China

We have reliable capacity estimates for 6 Chinese crania of *H. erectus,* 5 from Choukoutien and 1 from Lantian (Table 13).

Homo erectus OF CHOUKOUTIEN. The 5 most reliable determinations for crania of *H. erectus pekinensis* (Figure 29) would seem to be the following (Weidenreich 1943):

II	1030 c.c.
III	915 c.c.
X	1225 c.c.
XI	1015 c.c.
XXI	1030 c.c.

The mean for these 5 specimens is 1043 c.c., and the standard deviation, calculated from the range by the method for small samples, is very high, namely 133 c.c.—for the extreme range is large and the sample size small. It is a great pity that a new precise determination could not be attempted on the very large cranium with a capacity of 1225 c.c. The S.D. of 133 c.c. gives an estimated population range of 644 to 1442 c.c. on the basis of the sample mean plus and minus 3 S.D.s.

Homo erectus OF LANTIAN, SHENSI. This specimen was found in China in 1963. Its capacity was determined by Woo (1965), who used the biparietal endocast method proposed by me and yielded estimates for total capacity of 775 to 783 c.c. An estimate arrived at by the use of Pearson's formula was 778 c.c. Thus, Woo accepts the figure of 780 c.c. for the cranium. This

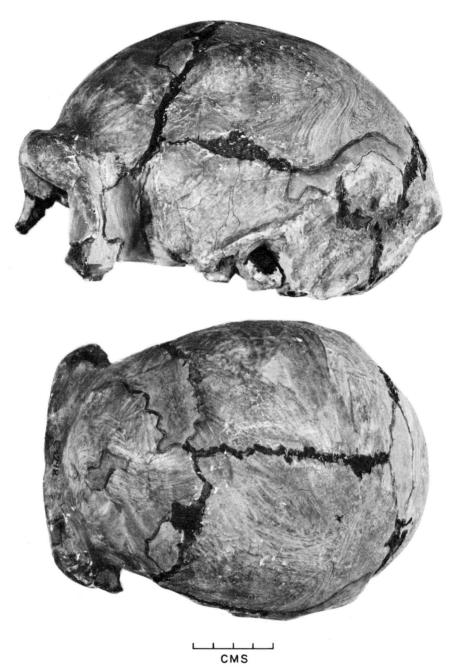

CMS

FIGURE 29: Norma lateralis and norma verticalis of the cranium of *Homo erectus pekinensis* III from Choukoutien, China. Its endocranial capacity, given as 915 c.c., is the smallest value recorded for the Choukoutien specimens of *Homo erectus,* though the Lantian cranium from Shensi is estimated to have had a capacity of only 780 c.c.

value is much lower than any of those from Choukoutien and, for this reason, as well as because of a number of other morphological traits, Woo has suggested that the Lantian specimen is closer to the Indonesian *H. erectus* IV from the Djetis Beds.

Summary on Asian Homo erectus

All of the foregoing Asian specimens (Table 13) are regarded today as belonging to a single species, *H. erectus,* although there may well be subspecific differences among them. Certainly, time differences seem to separate them. Perhaps, while we regard them as belonging to the same species, we should recognize the existence of an earlier, smaller-brained subspecies or race and of a later, larger-brained race. Even this division is not clearcut, because of the large area of overlap between the estimated population ranges of the Javanese and Pekin forms.

The mean for all 12 Asian crania of *H. erectus* is 929 c.c. The mean for the Indonesian group is some 70 c.c. less and for the Choukoutien group some 114 c.c. more than this value.*

Cranial capacity of African Homo erectus

I have excluded as African representatives of *H. erectus* the crania of Broken Hill and Hopefield (Saldanha), which Coon (1963, p. 337) would classify as *H. erectus.* Of the northwest African fossils attributed to *H. erectus* (and formerly designated *Atlanthropus mauritanicus*), none has provided an estimate of the cranial capacity. The only *H. erectus* specimen from Africa that has allowed a reasonable estimate of the endo-cranial capacity is the magnificent cranium, Olduvai Hominid 9, from the upper part of Bed II (Figure 30). Assisted by A. R. Hughes, I determined the capacity as 1000 c.c (Tobias 1965b, 1965c, 1967a). This value falls almost exactly midway between the largest and smallest capacities determined for 12 Asian crania (750 to 1225 c.c., giving a midvalue of 987.5 c.c.)

Summary on Homo erectus

The total sample range for 13 crania of *H. erectus,* irrespective of geographical origin, is thus 750 to 1225 c.c., and the mean for the sample

* If the capacity of *H. erectus* VIII from Sangiran is included, the mean for 13 Asian crania of *H. erectus* is 937 c.c. The Indonesian group has a mean 54 c.c. lower and the Choukoutien group a mean 106 c.c. higher than this value.

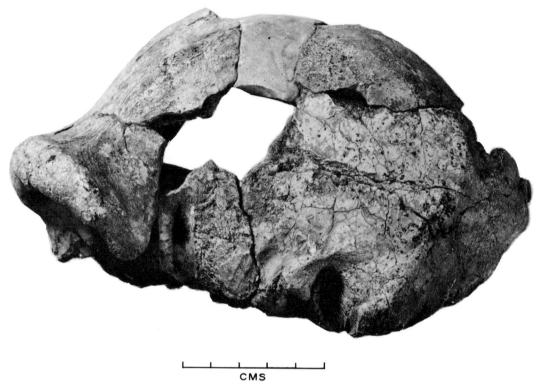

FIGURE 30: Cranium of Olduvai hominid 9, which is the best African representative so far found of *Homo erectus*. Its capacity has been determined by A. R. Hughes and me as 1000 c.c.

of 13 capacities is 935 c.c. (Table 13). If an estimate is made of the standard deviation on the basis of this range, it amounts to 142 c.c. On the assumption that the available sample lies in the middle reaches of the distribution for the total population, 3 standard deviations below and above the sample mean give an estimated population range of 509 c.c. to 1361 c.c.* This immense span covers the upper part of the australopithecine sample range, the entire *H. habilis* sample range, and the lower part of the *H. sapiens* range. With a difference of 852 c.c. between the lower and upper limits of the estimated population range, we see an extreme range almost as great as that which characterizes modern man, commonly cited as 1000 to 2000 c.c.

* With the inclusion of *H. erectus* VIII from Indonesia, the mean for a total sample of 14 crania becomes 941 c.c. and the estimated standard deviation 137 c.c. On this basis, the estimated population range would be 530 to 1352 c.c.

We should, however, be cautious before accepting this estimate of population range. There seems to be little doubt that between the australopithecine and habiline stages on the one hand, and the *H. sapiens* stage on the other hand, the mean cranial capacity of mankind doubled its size—from the 450 c.c. and 650 c.c. of the earlier stages to the 1300 c.c. and more of the sapient stage. The process of doubling the brain size is what characterized that stage of mankind usually lumped into the taxon *Homo erectus*. It is clear that selection must have been operating most vigorously in favor of larger brains during the emergence and life-span of the species *Homo erectus*. One might expect, therefore, that some populations of *H. erectus* would be characterized by appreciably larger brains and others by appreciably smaller brains than the species average. Two such populations may be represented by the Indonesian group (often recognized as the subspecies *H. erectus erectus*), with a sample mean capacity of 859 c.c., and by the Choukoutien group *(H. erectus pekinensis)*, with a sample mean of 1043 c.c. In relation to such subspecific groups, the position of the isolated specimens from Lantian and Olduvai must, for the time being, remain in suspense.

Under these conditions of a dramatic selection for larger brain size, with consequent diversification of populations with respect to this parameter, it may well be inquired whether it is biologically meaningful to compute a species average for the parameter in question and, by the pooling of data from such disparate populations, to attempt to assess the species standard deviation and population range. Statistically impeccable though the procedure might be, it may seriously be questioned whether normal statistical procedures can be invoked here under conditions of rapid evolution and changing patterns of brain size. The very meaningfulness of the biological events occurring at this critical stage of hominization may be masked by the statistical pooling of all the data from the geographically, chronologically, and evolutionarily dispersed populations.

NOTE TO CHAPTER FIVE

Professor Georges Olivier, head of the Laboratoire d'Anthropologie biologique in Paris, has used a somewhat different approach to estimate the standard deviations and population limits of hominoids (1971, personal communication). He based his estimate on Sacchetti's (1942) demonstration that there is an allometric relation between a dimension and its standard deviation and on Pineau's (1965) finding that the parameters fluctuate according to the nature of the measurements. "In the case of cranial capacities, a linear relation appears if the standard deviations proposed by Tobias are put into logarithmic co-ordinates." The slope of the line indicates that "the variability of cranial capacity increases faster than the absolute value of this measurement." Olivier has redrawn the allometric line using his own estimate of 1366 c.c. and 150 c.c. for the mean cranial capacity and standard deviation, respectively, of modern man. This permits him to read off standard deviations for the australopithecines (48 c.c.), *Homo habilis* (63.8 c.c.), *H. erectus* of Indonesia (91.2 c.c.), and *H. erectus* of China (114.8 c.c.). To compute population parameters, he considers that it would be injudicious—because the S.D. values are imprecise—to use the mean ±3 S.D.s. "It is sufficient to use the mean ±2 S.D.s to cover the normal biological variation, including 95 per cent of the subjects." By this method, and employing the mean capacities I published in 1968, Olivier arrives at the following variation amplitudes of hominid cranial capacities:

Population	Mean	Range
Australopithecines	500 c.c.	405–600 c.c.
Homo habilis	639 c.c.	510–770 c.c.
"*Pithecanthropus*"	880 c.c.	700–1060 c.c.
"*Sinanthropus*"	1075 c.c.	845–1305 c.c.
Modern man	1370 c.c.	1070–1670 c.c.
Classic Neandertal	1470 c.c.	1145–1795 c.c.

SIX

CRANIAL CAPACITY FROM AUSTRALOPITHECUS TO HOMO SAPIENS

Cranial capacity and hominid taxa

We have been led to conclude that the most startling jumps in brain size occurred with and after the emergence of *H. erectus*. The jump from the *A. africanus* mean of 494 c.c. to the *H. habilis* mean of 656 c.c. is of the same order of size as the jump from the mean for the Indonesian group of *H. erectus* (859 c.c.) to the Pekin group of *H. erectus* (1043 c.c.).

TABLE 14: *Jumps in cranial capacity from Australopithecus to Homo erectus*

A. africanus (if $\bar{x} = 494$ c.c.) to *H. habilis* (if $\bar{x} = 656$ c.c.)	162 c.c.
A. africanus (if $\bar{x} = 494$ c.c.) to *H. habilis* (if $\bar{x} = 668$ c.c.)	174 c.c.
A. africanus (if $\bar{x} = 442$ c.c.) to *H. habilis* (if $\bar{x} = 656$ c.c.)	214 c.c.
A. africanus (if $\bar{x} = 442$ c.c.) to *H. habilis* (if $\bar{x} = 668$ c.c.)	226 c.c.
H. habilis (if $\bar{x} = 656$ c.c.) to *H. erectus erectus* ($\bar{x} = 859$ c.c.)	203 c.c.
H. habilis (if $\bar{x} = 668$ c.c.) to *H. erectus erectus* ($\bar{x} = 859$ c.c.)	191 c.c.
H. erectus erectus ($\bar{x} = 859$ c.c.) to *H. erectus pekinensis* ($\bar{x} = 1043$ c.c.)	184 c.c.

Table 14 shows the intervals in the series of group means. It is interesting to note that the jump from the small sample of *H. habilis* ($n = 2$ or 3) to that of *H. erectus erectus* ($n = 6$, excluding Lantian) is only slightly more than that from the Indonesian to the Choukoutien groups of *H. erectus*. Yet the latter 2 groups are recognized as belonging to the same species! In other words, the difference in mean cranial capacity between 2 subspecies within *H. erectus* is only slightly smaller than that between the smaller-brained of the 2 subspecies and the *habilis* group, which some regard as a different genus (*Australopithecus*), from *H. erectus*. This underlines my contention that the rate of increase of brain size itself accelerated with the emergence and subsequent evolution of *Homo erectus*.

Figure 31 attempts to depict this rising tempo of encephalic increment from taxon to taxon.* It is of interest that the sequence corresponds roughly to the passage of time. Thus, while *A. africanus* and *H. habilis* overlap in time, it seems that the latest *H. habilis* populations outlasted the latest *A. africanus*. The evidence from Olduvai and from the Transvaal sites suggests that *A. africanus* was essentially a Lower Pleistocene (and probably, too, an Upper Pliocene) phase of hominid life; *H. habilis* was a Lower Pleistocene phase which apparently lasted into the earliest part of the *Middle Pleistocene* (as represented by Olduvai Bed II just above the faunal break). *H. erectus erectus* seems to have lived from the earliest to early Middle Pleistocene; *H. erectus pekinensis* perhaps in the middle part of the Middle Pleistocene; and *H. sapiens* from later Middle Pleistocene to Upper Pleistocene. These times are only approximate, for there is no clear and universally applicable definition of the boundaries between the different stages of the Pleistocene,

* Figure 31 does *not* take Holloway's (1970b) new estimates for *Australopithecus* nor Sartono's new *H. erectus* VIII into account.

97

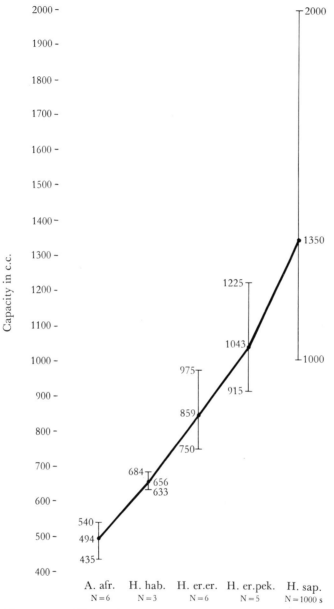

FIGURE 31: Tentative graphical representation of the increase in brain size from fossil to modern hominids. For each taxon shown, the sample mean and sample range are given. (A. afr.) *Australopithecus africanus;* (H. hab.) *Homo habilis;* (H. er. er.) *Homo erectus erectus;* (H. er. pek.) *Homo erectus pekinensis;* (H. sap.) *Homo sapiens.*

while the provenience of some of the relevant fossils is imperfect. Nevertheless, the general sequence of taxa shown corresponds approximately with the time sequence.

Cranial capacity and the time dimension

If we classify endocranial capacity according to the time dimension, we see that no Lower Pleistocene hominid specimen thus far recovered exceeded 685 c.c.

Lower Pleistocene hominids: * 435 (428), 480 (435), 480 (485), 500 (428), 540 (440), 500 (530), 530 (436), 530, 633, 684

Middle Pleistocene hominids (earlier and middle): 652, 750, 775, 780, 850, 890, 915, 915, 975, 1000, 1015, 1029, 1030, 1030, 1225

At the same time, no Middle Pleistocene hominid had a capacity lower than 650 c.c. In the above list I have included the Swartkrans specimen with the Lower Pleistocene hominids: Cooke (1963, p. 103) has stated that it is very likely that the Swartkrans and Kromdraai faunas "are close to the Villafranchian-Cromerian boundary, but it is still not certain on which side they lie." That is to say, it is not certain whether they are from the Lower or Middle Pleistocene. Since Swartkrans seems to be older than Kromdraai, it would seem reasonable to put the Swartkrans specimen among the Lower Pleistocene group.

It is not suggested that these sample limits tally with the population limits at any one time. Our estimates of standard deviations and ranges for the population have already shown that this is not so. Nonetheless, the samples may provide us with some evidence for a trend.

In brief, the proposition is suggested that during the latter part of the Lower Pleistocene, conditions of life became such that strong selective pressures for an increase in brain size became evident. The effect of such selection became manifest with the emergence of the larger-brained group known as *H. habilis,* but more emphatically with the arising of the next major systematic category, *H. erectus.*

We shall consider below what aspects of the life of *Homo habilis* and, especially, of *Homo erectus* could have been relevant for these selective pressures toward increasing brain size—factors such as the rise of systematic stone tool-making, organized and systematic hunting, and symbolic behavior including symbolic speech.

* Holloway's (1970b) reestimates are cited in parentheses.

The surmounting of a peak

Another provocative factor that arises on contemplation of the data on increasing capacity is that the selective pressures that led to the emergence and further development of the brain size of *Homo erectus* did not lapse. They did not lead to a graphical plateau in the heyday of *H. erectus*. The trend of rising mean endocranial capacities during the earlier stages of Pleistocene hominization undoubtedly continued into the Upper Pleistocene; it is reflected by a further increase in brain size in the early stages of *H. sapiens*.

Then the selective pressures seem to have relaxed somewhat, a few score thousand years ago (von Bonin 1934, Weidenreich 1946). Skulls of that date from Neandertal men of Europe, and also those of fossil men from Africa, had bigger braincases on the average than those of their present-day descendants. The graph of rising brain size flattened out to a plateau and then began to drop somewhat.

Although no attempt will be made here to review the evidence for this latest phase of hominization, some examples of Upper Pleistocene endocranial capacities from Africa may be quoted: Hopefield (Saldanha) ca. 1225 c.c.; Broken Hill 1280 c.c.; Gamble's Cave 1470 c.c. and 1530 c.c.; Naivasha 1453 c.c.; Taforalt 1376 c.c. and 1647 c.c.; Boskop 1650 c.c.; Fish Hoek 1550 c.c.; Matjes River crania 1230 to 1660 c.c.; and Asselar 1520 c.c. Most of the crania cited have high capacities, probably well above the mean for most present-day populations. This underlines the general statement made earlier that modern man—whether in Africa or Europe—would seem to have somewhat lower mean brain sizes than his forebears of the early Upper Pleistocene.

It seems that the trend toward increased brain size, which marked the first 2 or 3 million years of human evolution, had spent itself—and had done so as recently as the late Pleistocene. The wave of brain expansion had passed its peak. Some of our Stone Age men carried the twin processes of reduction of teeth and jaws, on the one hand, and expansion of brain, on the other, so far that they seem to represent an ancient foreshadowing of the popular idea of the man of the future. The matter has been most vividly portrayed by Loren Eiseley, Benjamin Franklin Professor at the University of Pennsylvania. In one of the essays in his delightful florilegium of anthropological sketches, *The Immense Journey,* he writes:

One . . . skull lies in the lockers of a great metropolitan museum. It is labelled simply: Strandloper, South Africa. I have never looked longer into any human face than I have upon the features of that skull. I come there often, drawn in spite of myself. It is a face that would lend reality to the fantastic tales of our childhood. There is a hint of Wells's Time Machine folk in it—those pathetic, childlike people whom Wells pictures as haunting earth's autumnal cities in the far future of the dying planet.

Yet this skull has not been spirited back to us through future eras by a Time Machine. It is a thing, instead, of the millennial past. It is a caricature of modern man, not by reason of its primitiveness but, startlingly, because of a modernity outreaching his own. It constitutes, in fact, a mysterious prophecy and warning. For at the very moment in which students of humanity have been sketching their concept of the man of the future, that being has already come, and lived, and passed away. [Eiseley 1958, 127–28]

When Eiseley shows his students in Philadelphia a picture of what the man of the future may be expected to look like, they say, "It's O.K. Somebody's keeping an eye on things. Our heads are getting bigger and our teeth are getting smaller. Look!" Eiseley continues:

Their voices ring with youthful confidence, the confidence engendered by my persuasive colleagues and myself. At times I glow a little with their reflected enthusiasm.

I should like to regain that confidence, that warmth. I should like to but. . . .

There's just one thing we haven't quite dared to mention. It's this, and you won't believe it. It's all happened already. Back there in the past, ten thousand years ago. The man of the future, with the big brain, the small teeth.

Where did it get him? Nowhere. *Maybe there isn't any future.* Or, if there is, maybe it's only what you find in a little heap of bones on a certain South African beach.

Many of you who read this belong to the White race. We like to think about this man of the future as being White. It flatters our ego. But the man of the future in the past I'm talking about was not White. He lived in Africa. His brain was bigger than your brain. His face was straight and small, almost a child's face. He was the end evolutionary product in a direction quite similar to the one anthropologists tell us is the road down which we are travelling. [Ibid., pp. 129–30]

When one takes a long-term evolutionary look at this problem, it seems that a larger brain size may once have been vitally important in aiding survival—for instance, in a world teeming with wild animals and devoid of harnessed fire. The further development of man would seem to have placed less and less of a premium on the size of his brain. For culture and the benevolence of social life have taken the place of nimble wits as an insurance policy against extinction. Beyond a certain stage in the increase of brain size, we have no evidence that further increase in any way improved man's adaptive abilities.

TABLE 15: *Some extreme brain weights/capacities in well-known modern men*	1000–1100	Franz Joseph Gall
		Léon Gambetta
	1282	Walt Whitman
	ca. 1900	Daniel Webster
		Ivan Turgenev
		Dean Swift
		Otto Von Bismarck
	ca. 2200	Oliver Cromwell
		George Gordon, Lord Byron

We have reached a stage in human evolution—and I am convinced we reached it thousands of years ago—where 100 people with smaller brains stand just as good a chance of surviving to child-bearing age as 100 with larger brains, and are likely to leave no fewer children than the others. Brain size is no longer a yardstick to survival as it may once have been. We have used these very brains to create conditions in which mere brain size is of negligible importance; we have used them to develop new mechanisms of adaptation, tools, shelters, clothing, fire, social institutions—and central heating, air-conditioning, refrigeration, disinfection, mink coats, and sun-shades. You can have these things with a size $5\frac{3}{4}$ hat or with a size $8\frac{1}{2}$, just as it makes no difference what size shoe you take.

Within very wide tolerance limits, brain size seems to make no differ-ence as to your ability to avail yourself of the joys and benefits of modern living. So, too, it seems that brain size does not limit your ability to con-tribute to society, culture, science. Some gifted people, such as Léon Gam-betta and Franz Joseph Gall, have had very small brains. Others, also gifted, have had very large brains. Doctor Samuel Johnson had about 2000 gm., while Lord Byron and Oliver Cromwell had about 2350 gm. (Table 15). And some very ordinary persons have had equally large brains.

Small wonder that in 1963 Gerhardt von Bonin could say: "Certainly, the weight of the brain is a very poor indicator of its functional value" (von Bonin 1963, p. 42), and, again, "brain size as such is a very poor indicator of mental ability" (ibid., p. 76). A century earlier, James Hunt had stood before the Anthropological Society of London and declared, ". . . we now know that it is necessary to be most cautious in accepting the capacity of the cranium as any absolute test of the intellectual power of any race" (Hunt 1863, p. 13).

In the parlance of the evolutionary biologist, the selective pressures that once placed a considerable premium on big brains have somewhat relaxed since the late Pleistocene. Whatever advantages a larger cranial capacity must earlier have imported were no longer evident. It was no longer a key to survival to have a large, well-filled braincase.

The relaxation of the selective pressure, the reversal of the age-old trend toward increased brain size, casts into strong relief the other side of the coin. What was the advantage in having an increased brain size? Why did selection in favor of larger brains continue for as long as it did, and why did it seem to operate more energetically at some stages than at others? What is the neurological basis of increasing brain size? And what are its microscopic and physiological counterparts? The ensuing part of this book will be devoted to exploring some of these questions, although it will not presume to offer adequate and conclusive answers.

SEVEN

 # THE STRUCTURAL MEANING OF VARIATIONS IN BRAIN SIZE

On the perils of palaeoneurohistology

One is least qualified to speak on the palaeohistology of the hominid brain. On theoretical grounds brains may become larger from any one or any combination of the following factors: (a) more nerve cells; (b) bigger nerve cells; (c) more neuroglia; (d) more nerve processes; (e) longer nerve processes; (f) thicker nerve processes (thicker myelin sheaths); (g) more highly-branched nerve processes. These are 7 variables that may affect the total quantity of brain tissue alone. At any one moment in time, within a single species, are larger brains larger predominantly because they possess more neurons? Or are larger brains larger through a combination of any 2 or more of these 7 possible variables?

We simply do not know the answers to these questions for modern human brains within the range of normality. We shall see in a moment that we have a little more information when it comes to comparisons between different animals of different average brain sizes. But within our species we do not know what the microscopic or cellular basis is of varying brain size.

103 🪶

If we do not know that simple *physico-physical correlation,* how can we hope to make meaningful statements about the correlation between gross brain size and cellular structure on the one hand, and about psychical and behavioral attributes on the other? For the *physico-physical* correlation is basic to the *physico-psychical* association. We do not have the requisite information at either level.

Holloway (1968a, p. 145), moving outside the human species, has concluded that: "Gross size of the brain alone does not explain differences of behavior within the primate order." He is at pains to point out that

such correlations [as between brain-size and specific behavioral traits like memory, insight, forethought, symbolization] are not *causal* analyses, and that a parameter such as brain weight in grams, or volume in ml, or area [of cortex] in sq. mm, cannot *explain* the differences in behavior which are observed. [Ibid., p. 125; italics mine]

A more encompassing theory, Holloway states, should entail not merely the changes in brain size that have occurred in evolution but the internal reorganization of the cellular material of the brain. It is precisely at this level that we are most ignorant.

If we compare different species of mammals, many studies have demonstrated that larger brains are correlated with clearly defined cellular and chemical features. For instance, the bigger the brain, the lower is the density of nerve cells in that brain (Nissl 1898; von Bonin 1948; Tower and Elliott 1952; Shariff 1953; Tower 1954). Further, it has been claimed that neurons are bigger and nerve cell processes longer and more complex in bigger brains. The glia/neuron ratio is likewise higher. The claims and their validity have been well-summarized by Holloway (1968a). As he points out, an increase in dendritic branching means more synapses and more connectivity, and with this goes more complex behavior.

By this kind of analysis of different species increase in brain size is coming to be meaningfully analyzed in terms of its structural units. More complete knowledge of these units, in turn, may provide a more rational basis for understanding increasingly complex behavior. All this has been shown to apply in a series of living forms that are assumed to represent an evolutionary progression from one form to another up the scale. To a lesser extent, similar changes have been shown to apply to the ontogenetic development of individuals within a species. For the adult level, however, I reiterate the view expressed earlier: we do not have any clear picture of the histological and chemical differences between large and small brains among members of the same species. Therefore, we cannot pinpoint any cellular and chemical differences between large and small brains that would indicate a basis for different behavior. *Are* there differences in behavior and in achievement between individuals with big brains and individuals with small brains? Evidence for such differences does not seem to exist.

We must confess our ignorance of the functional meaning and value of different sized brains in modern human individuals.

If we are ignorant of these essential facts about varying brain size in modern man, our ignorance in relation to the interpretation of fossil man is even more abysmal. It is so for 2 main reasons: first, we can never know what the palaeoneurohistology of any early hominid was. (Only the now classical and curious case of the Gánovče endocast from Czechoslovakia may be cited in parenthesis: it was once seriously claimed of this specimen that it was a true fossil brain and not an endocast, and that impressions of the nerve cells could still be detected. Happily, the most recent account of the specimen treats it as an ordinary endocast–Vlček 1969.) Any statements we may make about the course of the probable changes in neural make-up from, say, *A. africanus* to *H. habilis,* or from *H. habilis* to *H. erectus,* would be purely by analogy and deduction. Such statements could never eliminate an element of conjecture and even speculation.

The second difficulty is that, with endocasts, we are dealing not with a replica of the brain but with an impression of the interior of the braincase. Therefore, the external form and size of the cast reflects the sum total not only of all the neural and glial factors listed above but also of a further set of variables, namely: (a) the thickness and volume of the pachymeninx or dura mater; (b) the thickness and volume of the leptomeninges, the arachnoid and pia mater, as well as of the subarachnoid space; (c) the volume of the cerebrospinal fluid; (d) the total bulk, thickness, and ramifications of the cerebral and cerebellar arteries meandering over the surface of the brain; (e) the caliber of the cranial venous sinuses, and the size of the cerebral veins and lateral lacunae of the superior sagittal sinus; and (f) the thickness of the cranial nerves, at least that part of them from their attachment to the brainstem to their disappearance into various foramina and bony canals.

This gives us another 6 variables to add to the previous 7. Thus, when studying endocasts, we are further removed from the detailed organization of the brain. And, a fortiori, we are still further removed from understanding the structural basis of behavioral differences and behavioral evolution.

Yet, the stony silence of an endocast has not daunted a number of workers from drawing inferences from the comparative and developmental fields. At the crudest level, such studies have related the size of the brain to the size of the body, of the orbit or eyeball, of the foramen magnum, of the spinal cord, or of various other bodily features.

Brain size and body size

A study of the size of the brain in relation to body size has been employed chiefly in comparisons between species, in an effort to show how preeminent the brain has become in man. It was Cuvier who first introduced the concept of relative brain weight, that is, the weight of the brain expressed as a fraction of the weight of the body (Krompecher and Lipak 1966). Cobb's picture of a small human female standing alongside a rhinoceros shows graphically the difference in relative sizes of brains. The woman may have a brain weight of 1200 gm. in a body weighing, say, 45 kg., whereas the rhinoceros has a brain that may weigh 600 gm. in a body of about 2000kg. (Cobb 1965). The brain/body ratio in the rhinoceros is 1:3300 in such a case; that of the woman is 1:38. Even more revealing is a glance at a *Brontosaurus,* one of the great dinosaurian ruling reptiles, perhaps 65 feet long, that lived in the Jurassic period: its brain constituted a mere 1/100,000th of its 35-ton bulk. A whale has a brain/body weight ratio of 1:10,000; an elephant's is 1:600; a gorilla's is 1:200; and a man's is about 1:45 (Table 16).

But it is sobering to see that while man's exalted brain constitutes just over 2 per cent of his body weight, this percentage is surpassed by that of the lowly house mouse (2.5 per cent, or 1:40), the porpoise, with a 1:38 ratio, the marmoset, with a 1:19 ratio, and the delightful little squirrel monkey (*Saimiri*) of tropical America whose brain occupies 1/12th, or 8.5 per cent, of its body weight (Cobb 1965)! Because man, the sapient, did not come out at the top, it is not surprising that man, the vainglorious and the arrogant, has been searching ever since for a variety of strange indices that would place him unequivocally and unassailably on the highest branch of the tree of life. For example, when the length of the hypothalamus is expressed as a fraction of that of the cerebrum, man has the lowest fraction, and so comes out on top (Kummer 1961); when the weight of the spinal cord is expressed as a fraction of the brain weight, man has the lowest fraction, and so comes out on top (Latimer 1950; Krompecher and Lipak 1966); when the cranial capacity is related to the area of

	Mammals	Ratio
TABLE 16: *Ratio of weight of brain to weight of body in certain mammals and reptiles (after Cobb 1965)*	Squirrel monkey (*Saimiri sciutea*)	1:12
	Tamarin (*Leontocebus*)	1:19
	Porpoise (Dolphin) (*Phocaena communis*)	1:38
	House mouse (*Mus musculus*)	1:40
	Tree shrew (*Tupaia javanica*)	1:40
	Man (*Homo sapiens*)	1:45
	Ground shrew (*Sorex minutus*)	1:50
	Monkey (*Macaca mulatta*)	1:170
	Gorilla (*Gorilla gorilla*)	1:200
	Elephant (*Elephas indicus*)	1:600
	Sperm whale (*Physeter catodon*)	1:10,000

Reptiles	
Crocodile	1:5,000
Stegosaurus	1:30,000
Brontosaurus	1:100,000

the foramen magnum, man has the highest value, and still ends up on top (Radinsky 1967)!

All the indices I have cited have a certain though limited usefulness when comparisons are made between one species and another. However, few studies have seriously addressed themselves to this problem *within* the species of man.

Matiegka (1902) and Pearl (1905) claimed that in man brain weight varies with body weight and with body height. That is to say, they claimed to find that taller people and heavier people have larger brains. However, more recent workers have questioned the correlation claimed to exist between brain weight and body weight within the human species.

Pakkenberg and Voigt (1964) have made a more refined analysis on the brains of European subjects. They showed that the increasing brain weight with increasing body weight found by the earlier workers really results from the fact that people with high body weight are usually taller than average. The earlier workers had failed to correct for body height when evaluating the relationship between brain weight and body weight. When this correction was made, it was found that *brain weight depends significantly on body height but not on body weight* (Pakkenberg and Voigt 1964, p. 303).

Exactly the same results were obtained by Spann and Dustmann (1965) in a study of 1229 male and 632 female brains in the medico-legal institute at the University of Munich: brain weight rose with increasing stature, but no association could be determined between brain weight and body weight. In 1966, Schreider reanalyzed some old brain and body measurements made in Paris in 1865–1870 by Paul Broca, one of the great anatomists of the last century. Schreider found that between brain weight and body height there was a positive correlation coefficient of 0.26 for 224 males and 0.31 for 111 females.

Clearly, if one does not allow for the varying average body sizes of different populations, one may be misled into making false statements about the existence of real differences in average brain size among the populations compared. Thus, in the Raymond Hoffenberg Lecture of 1969 I showed that as yet no single study on the supposed differences between the mean brain weight of Negroes and of Caucasoids is valid because, among a number of other reasons, none of them has expressed or taken into account the height or stature measurements of the populations from which the brains were drawn (Tobias 1970). In my study I attempted an analysis in which stature was considered. This produced results suggesting that the differences among various racial or population groups are negligible, once allowance has been made for body size.

The studies on brain-body size ratio have spawned one interesting line of thinking that attempts to bridge the gap between brain size and neuronal contents. This we shall discuss now.

Brain size and neurons

In comparisons among different animals, K. S. Lashley (who gave the James Arthur Lecture in 1945) suggested that the total amount of brain material, expressed as a fraction of total body size, *"seems to represent the amount of brain tissue in excess of that required for transmitting impulses to and from the integrative centres"* (Lashley 1949, p. 33). Following up this notion, Jerison (1963) has demonstrated that brain size may be considered as 2 separate components: the first is directly related to the size of the body, and it is bigger in Primates with bigger body size, and vice versa. The other component seems to vary independently of body size; it comprises the "surplus" nerve cells that are present over and above those required for the satisfaction of immediate bodily needs. These "surplus" nerve cells, Jerison suggests, are available for response to the challenge of

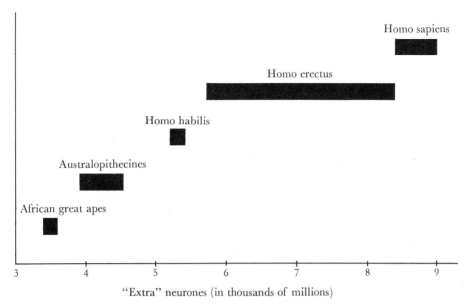

FIGURE 32: Numbers of "excess neurons" in hominoid brains, computed by Jerison's (1963) method. Small as are the samples available for australopithecines, *Homo habilis* and *Homo erectus*, the series shows a remarkable stepwise progression. Only the accumulation of more specimens and the refinement of the methods of analysis will verify whether the diagram represents a real evolutionary trend.

the environment through a wider range of brain-behavior mechanisms; that is, for intelligent adjustment.

On the basis of cell counts in a variety of Primates and, given certain assumptions, Jerison claims that it is possible to estimate the number of cortical nerve cells, not only in the brain as a whole but in each of the 2 components. He has developed a series of equations for the calculation of these neuronal values, given the size of the brain and the size of the body. By applying these formulae, he has been able to compute the number of "extra" neurons regarded as being available for brain-behavior adaptive mechanisms. With this second parameter, the number of "excess neurons," he has found it possible to differentiate various Primates, and especially the family of man, on the basis of the numbers of extra neurons. Modern man has far more excess neurons than, say, the chimpanzee and gorilla. While the African great apes can be shown by Jerison's equations to possess 2.4 to 3.6 billion excess neurons, modern man has 8 billion (Figure 32).

The method involves many assumptions. It does not adequately take into account regional variations in the density of neurons, in the ratio between neuroglia and neurons, in the size of nerve-cell bodies, and in the length and complexity of the dendritic processes of the neurons. Nonetheless, it provides a novel, approximate gauge of cortical development, which seems to go beyond the earlier intricate attempts of Eugene Dubois (1918a, 1918b, 1919, 1920, 1924, 1934, etc.) and others. Above all, the method has been developed for comparisons among species.

Table 17 conveys the results for a series of hominoids. The table gives a selection of measured endocranial capacities of individual specimens, or means of groups, estimates of body size in gm. or c.c., and then, derived from Jerison's equations, estimates of the total number of neurons in the whole brain and in that part of the brain related to body size, as well as the number of surplus or excess neurons.

A number of the figures in Table 17 are taken from Jerison's (1963) analysis. Others are based on my own computations or recomputations of capacities and body weights. Thus, for *A. africanus,* he based his estimate on a "brain size" of 500 gm. (which is close to the mean capacity of 494 c.c.) and a body size of 20,000 gm. I have recalculated these values for capacities of 500 c.c. (near the mean of published values), 435 c.c. (lowest published value in the sample) and 540 c.c. (highest value in the sample). The body weight of 20,000 gm. seems to be somewhat too small an estimate, and I have accordingly made the calculations for body weights of 25,000 gm. and 35,000 gm., associating the smaller brain sizes with the smaller body weight and the largest *A. africanus* capacity (540 c.c.) with the larger body weight. The estimates of "extra neurons" obtained by applying Jerison's formulae to these figures are 3.9, 4.3, and 4.5 billion, respectively; Jerison's figure for *A. africanus* fell near the upper end of this range of values.

Again, Jerison used a guess of 600 gm. for the brain size of *A. boisei* (formerly *Zinjanthropus*); I have used the value of 530 c.c., while adhering to his estimate of body size, namely 50,000 gm. This gave a value of 4.2 in place of his estimate of 4.7 billion.

Despite the altered values, and within the limitations of the method and the assumptions on which it is based, my results have corroborated one of Jerison's conclusions, namely that the australopithecines "were clearly, if only slightly, in advance of the level of brain evolution achieved by the anthropoid apes of our time" (Jerison 1963, p. 288). The pongid values range from 3.4 to 3.6 billion "excess neurons." *H. habilis* and *H. erec-*

TABLE 17: *Estimates of "extra neurons" in hominoids* [a]

	Measured endocranial capacity (in c.c.)	Estimated body size (in gms. or c.c.)	Estimates of total neurons (in thousands of millions)	Estimates of body-related neurons (in thousands of millions)	Estimates of "extra" neurons (in thousands of millions)
Chimpanzee	400	45,000	4.3	0.9	3.4
Gorilla A	540	200,000	5.3	1.8	3.5
Gorilla B	600	250,000	5.7	2.1	3.6
A. boisei	530	50,000	5.2	1.0	4.2 [b]
A. robustus	500	45,000	5.0	0.9	4.1 [c]
A. africanus	500	25,000	5.0	0.7	4.3 [b]
Taung ("adult value")	540	35,000	5.3	0.8	4.5 [c]
Sterkfontein 60	435	25,000	4.6	0.7	3.9 [c]
H. habilis (type)	680	35,000	6.2	0.8	5.4 [c]
H. habilis (paratype)	650	30,000	6.0	0.8	5.2 [c]
H. erectus	750	45,000	6.6	0.9	5.7 [c]
H. erectus	900	50,000	7.4	1.0	6.4
H. erectus	1000	50,000	8.0	1.0	7.0
H. erectus (range)	750–1225	50,000	6.6–9.4	0.9–1.0	5.7–8.4
H. sapiens	1300	60,000	9.5	1.0	8.5
Varied pop. means	1276–1400	53,000–68,000	9.4–10.0	1.0–1.1	8.4–8.9 [c]

[a] Modified and added to after Jerison 1963. [b] Recomputed for different brain or body size. [c] Own data.

111

TABLE 18: *Summary of "extra neurons" in hominoid taxa (in billions)*		
	African great apes	3.4–3.6
	Australopithecines	3.9–4.5
	H. habilis	5.2–5.4
	H. erectus	5.7–8.4
	H. sapiens (various populations)	8.4–8.9

tus could likewise be differentiated from the australopithecines on the one hand and from *H. sapiens* on the other: Jerison's figures for *H. erectus* were based on 2 specimens, the first of 900 c.c. and the other of 1000 c.c., which gave him values of 6.4 and 7.0, respectively. I have added the smallest *H. erectus* capacity thus far determined (750 c.c.) and a range for *H. erectus* from 750 to 1225 c.c., giving values ranging from 5.7 to 8.4 billion "extra neurons."

Similarly, the value for *H. sapiens* is given by Jerison as 8.5 billion; I have calculated outer limits of 8.4 to 8.9 billion for population means. The numbers of "excess neurons" are summarized in Table 18. It is of interest to note that the values for the type and paratype of *H. habilis* range from about halfway between those of the australopithecines and those of *H. erectus* to a point close to those of *H. erectus* (Tobias 1964, 1965c).

Holloway (1966, 1968a) has criticized Jerison's method, pointing out that his "mathematical extrapolations rest upon assumptions of cortical volume and neuronal density, and overlook the fact that in primate evolution, the cortex has undergone reorganization" (Holloway 1968a, p. 125). Further, Holloway has pointed out in the same place that Jerison's figures do not agree with the empirical counts made by Shariff (1953). On the other hand, Holloway has himself indicated elsewhere in the same paper (p. 142) that, "Actually, as Sholl (1956) has pointed out, Shariff's value for the volume of human cortex is somewhat low. . . ." Since Shariff's calculations of the number of neurons are based on neuronal densities *and on volume of cortex,* it is clear that if his estimates of the volume of the cortex are in error, so must be his computation of the number of neurons. Hence, the mere fact that Jerison's computation of the numbers of neurons differs from that of Shariff does not per se invalidate either Jerison's method or his results.

However, it is accepted that much more work needs to be done on the problems of neuronal densities, neuron size, length and complexity of branching, glia/neuron ratios—in different areas of the brain and at different ages, and in different living hominoids as well as lower Primates—and the results of such regional and other variations need to be taken into account in Jerison's approach before really significant and valid results may be deemed to have flowed from his method.

At any rate, it is gratifying to record that the slavish dependence on brain size *as a basis for interpreting behavior* is no longer so evident. That it is a *morphological* feature *in its own right* and worthy of study as such is undoubted. But the extent to which inferences as to behavior may be based upon it is very strictly limited. The attempt to look into the fossil brain by comparative and analytical and deductive means, such as rather courageous young palaeoneurologists like Jerison and Holloway are attempting, is most salutary. They are rising to the challenge posed in the closing words of von Bonin's little book, *The Evolution of the Human Brain* (1963), where he stated: "To write an evolution of the mind from the point of the view of the brain is not yet feasible."

Reorganization during the evolution of the brain

Several workers have recently stressed the major reorganization that the internal structure of the brain must have undergone during evolution to account for the differences encountered in living mammals and in Primate series. Few people have done more in recent years than R. L. Holloway Jr. to draw attention away from such traditional parameters as brain weight, cortical area, and even from such newer dissection instruments as are afforded by neuron density, neuron number, and glia/neuron ratios, and toward a probe into the patterns of structural organization that differentiate various living mammals and, especially, Primates (Holloway 1966, 1967, 1968a, 1969a, 1969b). Of course, he is not alone in this: von Bonin (1963, p. 77) has reminded us that "mere size completely leaves out of account the inner structure of the brain, which may be different in different forms and which may determine to a great extent what the brain can do."

Holloway has pleaded powerfully that the most important and, behaviorally, the most relevant internal changes during hominid brain evolution, including increase in brain size, are not the increased number of neurons (*pace* Jerison), nor changes in numbers and ramifications of processes, nor in glia/neuron ratios. Instead, the changes of greatest import for behavioral patterns are those involving *reorganization* of both cortical and subcortical components of the brain. It is unnecessary here to review all the evidence—comparative, experimental, and ontogenetic—bearing on such reorganization: in any event, a good deal of the evidence has been drawn together and summarized by Holloway (1968a).

Holloway's view may be summed up as follows: "The growth or expansion of cranial capacity is not our primary problem in understanding brain and behavioral evolution" (1970a, p. 309). Also: "Discussions of the brain in total mass must be replaced by more molecular appreciation of the range of structural and behavior changes for different extant primate species" (1968a, p. 165).

It may well be that he is correct. If so, our study of endocranial capacities will be simply a study of changing morphologies, but not of changing cerebral functions, nor of changing behavior patterns.

Interrelations of parameters

That the various sets of data are related, and causally related, is undoubted. Increase in brain size must have occurred together with increasing complexity of internal organization; increasing complexity of organization must have had its counterpart in changing functional patterns; these in turn permitted the emergence of changing patterns of behavior, as manifested, for instance, in material culture and hunting.

We know rather a lot about both ends of this causal chain: the size and shape of brain or endocast at one end; the cultural life and hunting behavior at the other end. It is the intermediate links in the chain that have eluded us up to now and that are becoming the object of serious investigation. The uncertainty of the intermediate steps by no means invalidates the study of the 2 termini of the causal chain.

In this volume I have thus far concentrated on one end of the chain, the endocasts. More particularly, I have concentrated on the total size as the most reliable parameter of the brain's or endocast's morphology. I have deliberately refrained from entering into a discussion of such features as the fissuration of the brain, because of the vagueness and uncertainty shrouding both the recognition and the interpretation of such fissural impressions on the endocranium and on the surface of the endocast. From his own studies and those that he made with Bailey, von Bonin (1963, p. 76) was driven to say forthrightly: "We consider the time and effort spent on the fissures of the fossil brains as largely wasted."

This review of the endocranial capacities of fossil hominids has left no doubt that a trend toward increasing brain size occurred from the earliest stages of hominid evolution reviewed here * to at least the penultimate stage, that of Upper Pleistocene man.

Not only is the trend manifest; one can go further and say that *it is the most strikingly sustained trend shown in the fossil record and, hence,*

---

* We have no data on the cranial capacity of the Mio-Pliocene creature, *Ramapithecus*, which, because of its teeth and jaws, is generally regarded today as a member of the Hominidae.

in the morphological evolution of the Hominidae. The rate, continuity, and duration of change in brain size seem on present evidence to exceed even those processes of dental and gnathic reduction that are such remarkable features of hominid evolution. The trend toward increased brain size is the most continuous, long-lasting, and marked hallmark of hominization.

Usually, when such a trend is detected in a fossil sequence, it is accepted that the feature in question has survival value. It is accepted that so sustained a line of development results from the operation of natural selection and that the feature in question is being positively selected. We may be inclined to say, therefore, that larger brain size must have conferred an undoubted advantage and that, down through the ages, larger-brained variants must have enjoyed greater opportunities for survival than smaller-brained ones.

What kind of advantages could a larger brain have conferred? We must assume that the larger brain incorporated more numerous and more intricately structured neural complexes, which permitted more complex functional patterns to be developed, which in turn endowed the organism with behavioral nuances and propensities, which equipped it better for survival to child-bearing age and reproduction. So, if we speak of the selective advantages of a bigger brain, we should add, "and all that went with it." For this is simply tantamount to saying that the selective advantage of the bigger brain resided in the nature of the behavioral patterns that the bigger brain made possible. The brain was not selected for its bigger size as such; the behavior patterns were selected—and it is just a convenient shorthand to say that bigger brains had survival value and were favored by natural selection. We *can* make such statements, even though we do not yet know all the intricate maze of systems that intervene between both ends of the chain, that is, gross brain size and behavior patterns. But we must never lose sight of the shorthand in which we are talking.

The chain of interrelations of parameters may be represented thus:

Increase in brain size

$\Updownarrow$

Increase in complexity of internal organization

$\Updownarrow$

Changing functional patterns

$\Updownarrow$

Changing patterns of behavior

Although we may agree with Holloway that the only studies that are really meaningful for behavioral interpretations are those that concentrate upon the intermediate links in such a chain, nevertheless the 2 ends of the chain remain valid objects of investigation in their own right.

Thus far, we have concentrated on one end of the chain, that of brain size, and have reviewed some of the attempts currently being made to probe beyond brain size to the underlying fine structure. Let us now approach the problem from the other end of the chain, that of behavioral traits, especially those of a cultural character.

EIGHT

 THE OTHER END OF THE CHAIN: THE CULTURAL CAPACITY OF PRIMATES

Cultural advancement is as striking a nonmorphological feature of hominization as increase in brain size is as a morphological yardstick. Bielicki (1969) has summarized the cultural traits or trait complexes "whose evolution has constituted the essence of hominization" as follows: (a) implemental behavior (tool-using and tool-making); (b) symbolic communication; and (c) certain characteristics of social organization, in which preagricultural human beings most markedly diverged from subhuman catarrhines (enumerated by Bielicki as "mating rules, home basis, within-group economic co-operation, sexual division of economic roles"—1969, p. 58). A further trait, namely hunting, Bielicki has classed among his list of "noncultural" features of hominization.

Of these 4 behavioral complexes, we have little evidence bearing on (b) and (c) and only some indirect evidence bearing on hunting. Item (a)— implemental behavior—is clearly the behavioral trait or trait-complex about which we have the greatest volume of material evidence.

Implemental activities among non-hominid Primates

When Dart (1926, 1929) first suggested that *Australopithecus* was capable of violent manual activities and of using and fabricating tools of bone, horn, and teeth (1956b), relatively little was known of the extent to which other higher Primates were capable of tool-using, and even to a certain extent of tool-making. Since that time more and more information has accumulated on Primate implemental activities. Proportionately, the resistance to attributing tool-using and tool-making activities to *Australopithecus* has waned. A brief review of the evidence from nonhuman Primates would therefore not be out of place.

The capacity for tool-using is widespread, not only in the great apes but also in lower Primates. Numerous reports tell of the use of objects as fighting tools as well as for nonagonistic purposes. These reports relate to behavior both in captivity and in the wild. For example, Bolwig (1961) reported on the tool-using activities of a captive olive baboon from the Sudan: these included purposeful throwing of sticks, the raking in of food beyond arm's reach, and the breaking of sticks to make a "ladder" with which to reach tidbits hanging overhead.

The remarkable feats of that clever little New World monkey, the capuchin, have been known at least since 1882, when G. J. Romanes reported the use by a brown capuchin monkey of the flat bottom of a dish to crack walnuts (cited by Weiner 1963). Klüver (1937) likewise reported on the capuchin's versatility and quickness in the use of a variety of differently shaped sticks, as well as of wire, rope, cardboard boxes, and other objects for obtaining food out of reach. Osman Hill (1960) has summarized the available evidence in the volume of his *Primates* series that deals with the Cebidae. A male capuchin in the London Zoo used a large marrow bone to crack open Brazil nuts and almonds when it was no longer able to do so with its teeth—which it had used when young (Vevers and Weiner 1963). We were able to confirm such behavior by a capuchin monkey in the Johannesburg Zoo: in the company of Dr. M. Lyall-Watson, then zoologist to the Zoo, and staff members and science students of the Anatomy Department, I observed 2 capuchins trying to open walnuts with their teeth; the first succeeded but the other failed. The second animal then laid the walnut on the floor of the cage, picked up a stone, and cracked the walnut open after a few well-aimed blows (Tobias 1965d).

Kortlandt and Kooij (1963) have reviewed what they describe as "Proto-hominid Behaviour in Primates." Analyzing a number of reports on agonistic throwing, scooping, clubbing, and stabbing by New and Old World monkeys and gibbons, they find these activities best developed in ground-living genera, such as baboons, and types that live predominantly in more open and diversified habitats, including rocky landscapes. Such behavior is less characteristic of more arboreal genera that live mainly in closed canopy

117 𝒴

forests; the only obvious exception to this rule is the capuchin. They concluded that, as with the great apes, a semiterrestrial life and a fairly open habitat in the wild tend toward the evolution of the genetic basis for the ability to perform aimed agonistic throwing, and/or for the actual inclination to do so in captivity. To this generalization the capuchin remains the exception.

Conversely, however, as Weiner (1963) pointed out, the tool-using abilities of a tree-living form such as the capuchin emphasize the point that a bipedal terrestrial mode of life per se is not a necessary preadaptation for the emergence of tool-using activities. He adds, though, that it must have been crucial for the change from tool-using to tool-making. On the basis of observations of higher Primates, we shall later have cause to question this latter view.

Abundant observations have now accumulated, not only on tool-using by the great apes but even on tool-fabricating. As Le Gros Clark stated in his Raymond Dart Lecture (March 1965), "it has now become clear that they [modern large apes with their small brains] are capable of more elaborate patterns of behavior than had hitherto been suspected."

The classical studies by Köhler (1924), Yerkes (1948), and others on chimpanzee behavior have in recent years been supplemented by a host of new studies. The facilities provided by the Witwatersrand University's Uganda Gorilla Research Unit enabled Donisthorpe (1958), Osborn (1963), and others to study the mountain gorilla; the most comprehensive studies on this ape have been made by Schaller (1963). The field studies of Kortlandt (1962) and of Jane Goodall (1963a, 1963b, 1964) have thrown much new light on the behavior of chimpanzees. These field researches have been supplemented by the zoo observations summarized by Kortlandt and Kooij (1963), the Hayes' experiments (1952) with Vike, Mrs. N. Kohts's (1935) experiments with her child's gorilla contemporary and playmate, and the exploration by Khroustov (1964) of the highest frontier of implemental activity in chimpanzees.

From this wealth of new information emerge certain key observations that bear on tool-using and tool-making or, if one prefers it, tool-modifying activities by the great apes. Tool-using activities—such as agonistic throwing, clubbing, and stabbing—characterize all 3 of the great apes—chimpanzee, gorilla, and orangutan—as Kortlandt and Kooij (1963) have well summarized. Nonagonistic uses by apes include isolated instances of branches being used by gorillas and one orangutan as raking tools for reaching fruit or other objects (Kortlandt and Kooij 1963). Beatty (1951) observed a chimpanzee pick up a rock and break open a dried palm nut. Merfield (1956) watched a group of chimpanzees poking sticks into an underground bees' nest and then licking off the honey. Kortlandt and Kooij (1963) reported the use of leaves as "medicated pads" by a chimpanzee and of small sticks and fruit as "toilet" aids by another chimpanzee.

Goodall saw chimpanzees use natural objects as tools on many occasions. For instance, she saw chimpanzees use sticks to feed on different species of ants (1964): the nests were opened, a stick was thrust in, left for a moment, and then withdrawn with the ant-mass on the end. The delicate morsel was licked off with the lips. Termite "fishing," however, provided her with one of her crucial observations. In those months (November to January, approximately) when the termites extended their passages to the surface of the nest, chimpanzees plucked stalks and small twigs, pushed them into openings on the surface of the termitarium, withdrew the tools, and picked off the insects with their lips. They would move away from the termite heap to pluck grass stalks, carry back one or even several, and settle down for an hour or two's peaceful "fishing." Sometimes tools were carefully prepared: leaves were stripped from stems or twigs with the hand or lips, and long strips were sometimes pulled from a piece of grass that was too wide. As the straw became bent at the end, the chimpanzee would break off the bent pieces until the tool was too short for further use. We have here evidence not only of the use of natural objects but also of their modification to render them more suitable for the purpose to which they are put (Goodall 1964).

Another form of rudimentary tool-fabrication consisted in the use of leaves as drinking tools. Chimpanzees would drink water from natural bowls until the level was too low for the water to be reached with the lips. Thereafter, leaves were stripped from twigs and chewed briefly, giving a crumpled surface. Then the leaf-mass, held between the index and middle fingers, was pushed into the bowl, withdrawn, and the water sucked out of it. The process was repeated until the bowl was empty or until the chimpanzee lost interest (Goodall 1964).

The cultural Primates

By modifying natural objects, the chimpanzee may be said to have reached the first crude beginnings of tool-making. Goodall has written:

It is unlikely that this practice of fishing for termites is an inborn behavior pattern. Among higher primates, behavior is found to depend more and more on learned techniques and less and less on "instincts." It seems almost certain that this method of eating termites is a social tradition, passed from ape to ape by watching and imitation. As such, it must be regarded as a crude and primitive culture. [Goodall 1963b, p. 308]

Kortlandt and Kooij (1963) would agree with this view. According to the laboratory experiments and zoo experience they have reviewed, the behavior of the great apes, unlike that of monkeys, is moulded largely by maternal education, social traditions, and other environmental factors, rather than by innate factors. "This applies," they point out, "to locomotion, nest building, food choice, sexual behaviour, social intercourse, etc., and, to some extent, even to maternal care" (1963, p. 61). Therefore, according to these workers, the great apes and man might be characterized as "cultural Primates," whilst the gibbons and monkeys would be classified as "instinctual Primates," provided that we may use the term "culture" for a nonverbalized system of social traditions. (Unfortunately, there exists no appropriate term to designate nonhuman, speechless culture.) (Ibid., p. 62.)

These primatologists thus align the apes with man because the behavior patterns of the apes are largely learned rather than genetic or instinctual. Of course, there is no sharp dividing line. There must be a smooth transition from the instinctual to the learned patterns of behavior, and even in modern man there is often doubt as to the degree to which he has thrown off instinctual patterns and substituted learned ones for them. However, Kortlandt's distinction between the cultural Primates and the instinctual Primates is a useful one. It is in line with other recent evidence tending to show a much closer relationship between the great apes (especially the African ones) and man. The new evidence includes data on the chromosomes and on the serum proteins of the apes. It seems that we must now add to the evidence of comparative anatomy not only that of cytogenetics and serology but also ethological evidence, that is, data drawn from the field of animal behavior.

The limits of implemental activities by apes

In an attempt to ascertain the limits of implemental activity possible in apes, G. F. Khroustov (1968) in Moscow devised an elegant series of experiments on chimpanzees. A food bait was placed in a metal tube of such diameter and length that neither the chimpanzee's fingers, toes, nor lips could reach the bait. Then, to get at the bait, the chimpanzee was faced with a series of situations of increasing complexity that made increasing demands of tool-using and tool-making for their solution. The experiments may be summarized as follows:

1. A straight smooth rod was provided, that is, an implement suitable for the action required. The chimpanzee had no difficulty in pushing out the bait.

2. The same rod was provided, but with a crosspiece at one end. The chimpanzee did not immediately find the correct solution. The idea that the stick had to be inserted into the tube had, apparently, fixed itself in the animal's mind—but no more than that, for it at first grasped the stick by the free end and attempted unsuccessfully to insert the end with the crosspiece into the metal tube. Later, it tried the other end with success. In both these preliminary experiments, success could be achieved without any modification of the tool.

3. In the third stage, some modification of the tool was necessary. The rod was fitted with 2 crosspieces, one at either end. After unsuccessful attempts to use the rod directly as an implement, the animal broke off one crosspiece: however, the earlier associations were not sufficiently fixed in its mind, and it then attempted to thrust into the tube the other end with intact crosspiece. Only after the failure of such attempts did the animal find the correct way to use the rod. It seems that the connection had not yet been established between the changes that it wrought on the implement and the possibility of using it as an implement. To quote Khroustov:

The destructive actions of the anthropoid on the one hand and its attempts to perform implemental action on the other remained separate operations not united into a chain. Only by establishing the connection between these operations and their organization into a single chain do the destructive actions receive definite direction, turning into a directed treatment of the implement and thus forming a link in the whole chain of activity. [Ibid., p. 505]

Further experiments led the chimpanzee to hit upon the connection that had escaped it before. It was given a tree branch with a side shoot: it broke off the shoot and so gained the bait with the branch. When it was again given the rod with 2 crosspieces, after some hesitation and several abortive trial-and-error actions, the connection seems suddenly to have been established. The chimpanzee grasped the rod, immediately broke off both crosspieces and the string binding them, and then used the free rod as an implement.

It seems that this stage fixed in the mind of the animal the idea of treating an object to adapt it for an action that the animal was trying to perform with its help.

Up through this stage of the study, the elements of the object were clearly manifest to the chimpanzee; but in ensuing experiments the features of the implement were progressively obscured.

4. The chimpanzee was provided with a long, thin, rectangular plate. In this case the material given was not structurally divided into a ready implement and elements that hindered its use. Now it was necessary for the animal to break the object: this it did in a variety of experiments, until one of the resulting fragments suggested the form of the original rod-shaped implement.

5. In the next experiment a circular disc of the same sort of wood was provided: thus, nothing was manifest of the form of the necessary implement. The animal was required to transform the disc into certain parameters, not on the basis of any indications on the disc but solely on the basis of information about them fixed in the mind of the ape. The chimpanzee proved equal to this task.

6. Before breaking the disc the chimpanzee turned it so that the grain lines of the wood ran away from its body. Hence, it was subsequently given discs with imitation grains drawn at right angles to the true grain. At first the chimpanzee began to operate according to the illusory grain; finding the disc difficult to break, it changed the direction of its actions and was successful.

7. The disguise was made more complete: grooves were *carved* on the disc at right angles to the grain of the wood. Both surfaces of the wood were then covered in thick paper, with the grooves forming a clearly discernible relief; furthermore, black lines were drawn between the furrows perpendicular to the grain. Again the illusory grain misled the chimpanzee. After repeated trials and errors it changed the direction and had success, assisted by using its teeth to make a number of consecutive dents along the true grain.

Khroustov concluded that "active transformation of material having a preliminary neutral form, despite its false outer appearances, into an implement with definite parameters, is a fully attainable stage of activity for a chimpanzee" (ibid., p. 506). In Khroustov's opinion, this is the level of implemental activity characteristic of the australopithecines. "Its coming into being signifies not the appearance of the human principle but a high stage of its functional preparation, which is a necessary prerequisite for the transition to the primary forms of labor, as an activity peculiar to human beings" (ibid., p. 507).

8. Finally, once the chimpanzee had mastered the full manufacturing of the implement under the conditions just outlined, further experiments were devised to find the limits of its experimental activity. A similar series of objects was given to the animal and it had to make the same implement. Only this time the rods and discs were of a tough wood, which the animal was unable to break with its natural equipment of hands, feet, and teeth. A stone implement in the form of a hand ax was provided to assist the chimpanzee in breaking the tough wood. Numerous and persistent attempts were made by the chimpanzee to break the wood, but in none did he try to treat the unyielding material with the stone implement, or with anything other than his natural or bodily equipment. For the first time in the whole series of experiments, an attempt was made by demonstration to teach the chimpanzee what he needed to do, namely to use the stone tool. Even then, the chimpanzee made no attempt to copy the actions of the experimenter and use the stone implement, despite its most strenuous and prolonged efforts after the demonstration to overcome the resistance of the material. It seems that the decisive step of *using a tool to make a tool* was impossible for the ape under these experimental conditions.

Whether an ape could overcome this barrier under other conditions can be determined only by further experiment. Meantime, Khroustov concludes that:

The limited scope of using the natural organs as means for making adaptational changes of implements tied down the development of the implemental activity of man's ancestors to definite boundaries and possibilities. When these were exhausted, the immediate forebears of man by force of necessity were brought to the threshold of the frontier, on the surmounting of which depended their survival. [Ibid., p. 508]

That is, they needed to learn to use objects as a means for transforming materials into implements—and so they crossed the frontier itself: "the creation of artificial means for producing implements" (ibid., p. 508).

Thus, using a somewhat narrower definition of human cultural behavior than that used by Kortlandt and Kooij, Khroustov draws a line between the apes and man and aligns the australopithecines in this regard with the apes.

It is clear that the level of implemental activity that the living great apes can attain in the wild, in captivity, and under experimental conditions far exceeds what had earlier been thought. These new bodies of information culled by specialists in Primate behavior have as yet scarcely made their impact upon the interpretation of archaeological problems and of australopithecine cultural potentialities. That is why I make no apology for having dwelt on them at such length here: for they must alter the climate of opinion in palaeoanthropology, and they must influence the way in which we consider the claims made for the australopithecines. In fact, the accretion of this new information in the last decade has been paralleled by a steady decline in the resistance to claims made about implemental activity of the australopithecines.

NINE

 THE CULTURAL CAPACITY OF AUSTRALOPITHECUS

Our discussion of the cultural potentialities of Primates has brought us directly to the basic questions: did *Australopithecus* have the capacity for tool-using and tool-making? If so, in what manner and in what directions did he use these capacities? Answers to these questions are provided by 2 main avenues of thought: indirect inference and direct evidence.

*Indirect evidence bearing on the cultural
capacity of Australopithecus*

Much indirect evidence points to the cultural adaptation of *Australopithecus* (Tobias 1965d, 1968c, 1969b). Such evidence stems from (a) the ecological situation in which australopithecine fossils have been found; (b) the possession by *Australopithecus* of the basic anatomical equipment required for implemental activity; and (c) the fact that *Australopithecus* was structurally advanced over the apes, especially in those respects relevant for tool-making.

THE ARGUMENT FROM ECOLOGY. Remains of *Australopithecus* have been found in areas of comparative aridity, as well as in somewhat moister climates. Climatological evidence, past and present, suggests that they were well adapted to life in open savannah country. In contrast, the African great apes are confined to the more sheltered environment of forest and woodland. It might be suggested that a ready wit, versatility, and inventiveness would be necessary for survival in the challenging environment of open country, with little natural protection from the carnivores and the elements. It is not reading too much into this ecological fact to suggest that, to survive in open country, the relatively defenseless *Australopithecus* would have had to depend on his wits and resourcefulness to a far greater extent than would an ape in forested terrain.

THE ARGUMENT FROM GENERAL BODILY STRUCTURE AND FUNCTION. The basic list of structural requirements for implemental activity comprises: (a) brains of sufficient quantity and quality; (b) a strong element of learned rather than exclusively or mainly instinctual patterns of behavior; (c) stereoscopic vision; (d) a prehensile hand capable of some degree of precision in gripping; and (e) freeing of the forelimbs for short or long periods, as in sitting upright.

These basic requirements are fulfilled in numerous middle and higher Primates; so that the anatomical potential for implemental activities is found in baboons, monkeys, gibbons, great apes, and man.

Moreover, all the items on this list of features that we can confirm from the fossil record are present in *Australopithecus*.

THE ARGUMENTS FROM SPECIFIC ANATOMICAL AND FUNCTIONAL FEATURES OF *Australopithecus*. *The teeth of Australopithecus*. All of the australopithecines differ from the pongids or apes in possessing relatively small canine teeth that do not project to any appreciable extent beyond the plane of the occlusal surfaces of the adjacent teeth (Robinson 1956; Tobias 1967a). The absence of large canines strongly suggests that *Australopithecus* must have used alternative mechanisms—manual and implemental—for solving those sorts of problems for which apes use their large canines.

The brain behind the hands. Although the mean capacity of the brain-case of *Australopithecus* is very similar to that of the gorilla, we have enough of the skeleton of the ape-man to indicate that his body weight was probably far less than that of the gorilla. In other words, his estimated brain/body weight ratio, or *relative brain size*, was higher than that of the biggest-brained species of the living great apes. Then, too, the external configuration of the brain of *Australopithecus* shows a number of manlike features. It would seem likely that a brain that is more hominized in size and shape is likewise more hominized in its fine internal structure necessary to permit the emergence of more complex patterns of behavior than those of the apes.

Upright posture. Australopithecus was essentially bipedal: he did not depend upon his hands in locomotion to the same extent as the apes. Likewise, when at rest, he undoubtedly possessed that widespread Primate habit of sitting upright with hands freed, while the structure of foot, knee, thigh, and pelvis indicates anatomical adjustments to upright stance. Thus, whether he was sitting, standing, walking, or running, the hands of *Australopithecus* were freed for long periods of time. Hands were thus available for manual and implemental activities for far more of the day than were those of other Primates whose hands were liberated only during the process of sitting upright. In contrast, the occasional, sporadic, and nonhabitual bipedalism of apes does not occupy any significant period of time within the day; it is of interest chiefly in indicating how widespread among the Primates is the capacity for uprightness, which only the hominids specialized in and made a part of their peculiar and specific adaptations.

Many are the views about the relationship between uprightness and tool-using and -making. But all agree that the capacity for implemental activity is at least enhanced by uprightness. If nothing else, the creature can spend more of its time on manual activities.

The hand. The attainment of uprightness meant the freeing of the hand. This, in turn, led to, or was accompanied by, a change in its structure and functioning. The hand became more capable of oppositional movements between thumb and other fingers than are the hands of apes, and so precision movements, as defined by Napier (1960), became anatomically more feasible, easier, and more precise. We have relatively few hand-bones of *Australopithecus*, namely a capitate (TM 1526) from Sterkfontein, 2 metacarpals from Swartkrans, and 1 from Kromdraai; in addition, from Olduvai we have a capitate, scaphoid, trapezium, and 6 metacarpals, all of which have been attributed to *Homo habilis* (Tobias 1971). These hand- and finger-bones show manual hominization, though to an imperfect degree.

SUMMATION ON STRUCTURAL HOMINIZATION OF *Australopithecus*. It is clear that *Australopithecus* was structurally more hominized than living, nonhuman, higher Primates, especially with respect to those features relevant for implemental activities.

We may conclude that the structural and functional potential for implemental and cultural capacity not only was present in *Australopithecus* but exceeded that of any of the extant apes. It may be inferred that anything a chimpanzee or a gorilla can do *Australopithecus* could have done—and probably could have done better! If a chimpanzee can "fish" for termites and make sharpened crowbars for opening banana-boxes, so could *Australopithecus* have done in a similar problem situation. If gorillas can make comfortable, sprung beds, so might *Australopithecus*. If chimpanzees can break a circular disc of wood to make a narrow stick with which to extract food from a cylinder, so too could *Australopithecus* have done in a similar problem situation.

This being so, all the evidence indicates that we should group *Australopithecus,* along with the great apes and man, among the "cultural Primates" as designated by Kortlandt and Kooij (1963). We should expect that *Australopithecus* could go even further than these very intelligent actions of the apes.

Hence, on ecological, anatomical, functional, and comparative grounds, there is a strong a priori case for *Australopithecus* having been a tool-user and -maker. Is this inference supported by any direct implemental evidence?

Direct evidence on cultural activities by
Australopithecus

As recently as 1964, Le Gros Clark wrote: "Practically nothing is known of the activities or mode of life of *Australopithecus*" (1964, p. 171). This seems to reflect a poor yield of facts forty years after the first discovery of *Australopithecus*. A closer look may, however, show us that, with due allowance for the uncertainties of all archaeological interpretation, we have reason to believe that we are approaching some knowledge and some understanding of the cultural life of *Australopithecus*.

CULTURAL OBJECTS OF BONE, HORN, AND TOOTH. Since our first excavations began at the australopithecine site of Makapansgat, 200 miles north of Johannesburg, some twenty-five years ago, we have kept every single specimen—including slivers and fragments—of fossilized bone developed from the tough matrix or breccia. We now have over 100,000 classified pieces of bone from this ape-man bearing site. A study of some of these specimens first convinced Dart (1956b, 1957) that many of them had been used as tools, perhaps in the same adventitious way that sticks and stones are used by higher Primates. Closer study revealed consistent patterns of breakage in many specimens. They suggested to Dart that not only had these bones been used as tools but they had been deliberately modified over and above their

127 ✘

original shape to provide better tools. This is not a far-fetched idea when we know that chimpanzees will whittle away the end of a stick to make a sharp point for prising, as in a crowbar, or will modify the form of a piece of wood to make a tool serviceable for solving problems. Yet Dart's claims, stated with his accustomed vigor, have aroused much opposition, especially from those who have not studied the original specimens. Some of his fellow scientists, it would seem, have been more ready to accept that *Australopithecus* made stone tools than that he modified and used a material readily at hand, namely the bones of the animals eaten—and this despite the fact that bone has formed an integral part of the cultural materials of man in every other culture from that of Choukoutien to the present.

A few points relevant to the bone-tools hypothesis are as follows:

1. The Makapansgat cave deposit contains mountainous accumulations of bone. The more than 100,000 pieces thus far collected represent a small fraction of the largely untouched in situ accumulations apparent in numerous exposures within the cave earth. No natural accumulations of bone by scavengers or predators have ever been found to equal this for sheer quantity.

2. Tooth-marks of hyena, leopard, and porcupine are conspicuously absent from all but a handful of the many thousands of bones.

3. Statistical analysis of the bones from the Makapansgat deposit has shown definite evidence that certain bones have been selected, and others neglected. Thus, the ratio of proximal to distal humeral fragments is less than 1 to 10, while the ratio of humeri to femora is over 5 to 1. Some selective agency has clearly been at work.

4. Large concentrations of ungulate humeri and other long bones show signs of damage inflicted before fossilization on the epicondyles or extremities.

5. Many of the bone objects can be classified in categories of recurring patterns, such as those that Dart has rather fancifully named daggers, scoops, pestles and mortars, and compound ripping tools. Whatever the names and whatever the uses that may be attributed to them, the fact remains that regular and consistent patterns do occur (Figures 33 and 34). Has anyone been able to demonstrate similar regularities and constant patterns among the bone debris of carnivores?

6. Many of the bone flakes show signs of differential wear and tear along one edge, or at one end, but not the other.

7. A number of special cases included horn-cores and smaller long

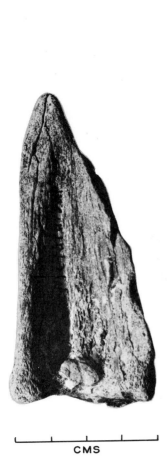

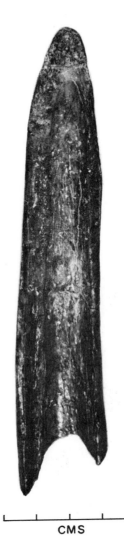

FIGURE 33: Bone point on part of
the shaft of an ungulate meta-
tarsal from Makapansgat.
There is a suggestion of facet-
ting on the left and right margins near the point.

FIGURE 34: Well-shaped bone point
made from half the split shaft
of a limb-bone from Makapansgat.

bones rammed and lodged up the marrow cavities of broken larger bones (Figure 35).

8. In several instances small bones and even stone flakes have been wedged between the condyles of long bones (Figure 36).

9. Numerous long bones show signs of having been broken by a kind of spiral torsional stress.

10. In one analysis 80 per cent of over 50 baboon crania from Taung (21), Sterkfontein (22), and Makapansgat (15) show signs of damage by localized violence—such as a single depressed fracture, or perhaps 2 adjacent ones. Some of the ungulate humeri have damaged epicondyles that fit some of the fracture depressions on the baboon crania.

11. There is some slight evidence of stone-collecting habits: a small number of quartz and quartzite pebbles and fragments have been found in the breccia.

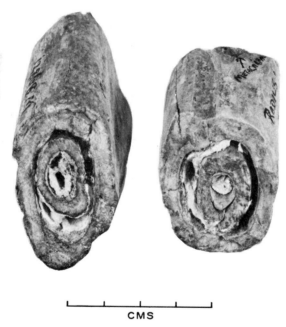

CMS

FIGURE 35: Shaft fragments of 2 antelope long bones from the grey breccia at Makapansgat. The left specimen shows a metacarpal wedged inside a tibia; at the far end, where the metacarpal widens toward its extremity, the inner bone is firmly impacted against the wall of the marrow cavity of the outer bone, with virtually no calcite intervening. The right specimen is of a metacarpal wedged up the marrow cavity of a radius.

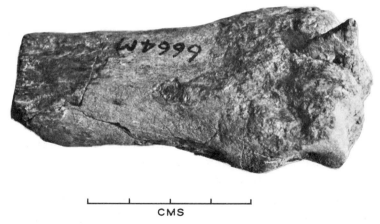

CMS

FIGURE 36: Oblique dorsal view of an antelope metacarpal with a triangular
flake of bone wedged in position in the deep cleft between the 2 condyles
of the bone.

12. Another material readily at hand—stalactite and stalagmite—has been
found broken off in the deposit, and some fragments were further fractured
transversely and longitudinally. Where is the carnivore that indulges in such
behavior?

It may well be inquired why comparable masses of what Dart calls
osteodontokeratic objects have not been reported from Taung or Sterkfontein, especially as there are numbers of fractured baboon crania at both sites.
At neither site can it be said that more than a fraction of the breccia has
been thoroughly searched for broken bone fragments other than taxonomi-
cally identifiable parts. Yet, Robinson has described a selectively polished
bone implement from Sterkfontein that, after a careful analysis for possible alternative causal agencies, he concludes "can only be explained as a
by-product of intelligent hominid behaviour" (1959, p. 585). Similarly,
L. S. B. Leakey (1960) has recorded "a genuine bone tool" from the site
F.L.K.N.N.I. (the type site of *Homo habilis*) in Olduvai Gorge. And his wife,
M. D. Leakey (1967), has recorded "a few bone fragments with evidence of
utilization" at sites of the "Oldowan Culture" in the lower part of the
Olduvai sequence. From M.N.K. and other sites in the middle and upper
parts of Bed II, she has described a number of bones "which had been arti-
ficially shaped and subsequently utilized" (M. D. Leakey 1967, p. 440).

Dart's standpoint may be restated thus: the simplest hypothesis that at
once explains all the above sets of facts about the Makapansgat bones is

that some primitive hominids, most likely *Australopithecus,* were responsible for the bone accumulations and had a well-developed cultural life based primarily upon the use and modification of bone. We know already that the manufacture of such artefacts was probably well within the somatic capacity of *Australopithecus.* No other single hypothesis can explain more than a proportion of the above facts. Occam's razor might well lead us to accept Dart's interpretation, if not in its full detail then in broad principle, as the most likely single explanation of the otherwise almost inexplicable mountains of bones at Makapansgat, with their selected, fractured, and patterned characteristics (Tobias 1968c).

It may, of course, legitimately be inquired whether it is necessary to assume a *single* explanation for the bone accumulations. Of course, it is not necessary to do so. Undoubtedly, such factors as rodent and carnivore activities also may have played a part—but the nature of the bone accumulations at Makapansgat is not such that the lion's share of the great bone concentrations there may readily be attributed to such factors. Water action, colluvial hill-wash, and accidental factors cannot be excluded as additional agencies. However, at Makapansgat, at any rate, the totality of evidence summarized above seems to point to hominid activities as being the most important agency responsible.

At one other site, Swartkrans, in the Transvaal, Brain (1968b, 1970) has produced evidence suggesting that carnivore activities, especially that of leopards, may have been responsible in the main for the accumulation of hominid material there. It is an interesting fact that hominid specimens occur at Swartkrans in greater numbers than at any other site; indeed, some 40 per cent of all the australopithecine and other early hominid material thus far discovered has emanated from Swartkrans (Tobias 1971). These special conditions may well demand a special explanation at that site, such as Brain's leopard hypothesis. However, the leopard hypothesis has been invoked to explain the presence there of such large numbers of hominid remains—including one with what appear to be leopard tooth-marks—but not, as I understand it, to explain the presence of bones in all other deposits. The leopard hypothesis for the Swartkrans hominid remains does not weaken the hominid hypothesis to explain most of the Makapansgat animal accumulations.

A preponderance of osteodontokeratic activities, such as are evidenced at Makapansgat, need not have characterized all early hominid populations of the Lower Pleistocene. The southern African australopithecines of the

Lower Pleistocene may have been an exceptional and atypical group for their time: their peripheral and ecologically difficult situation may have elicited—or retained—bone tool-making as one of several possible solutions to the challenge of their environment. In eastern Africa bone seems to have played a relatively minor role as a cultural solution resorted to by early Pleistocene hominids. There, at any rate, by about the same time, another solution—stone tool-making—had been adopted, very probably by somewhat more advanced hominids. The bone artefacts of Makapansgat may even represent the persistence in southern Africa of a yet earlier, possibly Mio-Pliocene, phase of cultural hominization—in much the same way as the African subcontinental cul-de-sac has so often preserved, and indeed still conserves, archaic species of animals long after their extinction in more northerly latitudes.

Indeed, Pilbeam and Simons (1965) have spoken of evidence, direct and indirect, for the existence of small-canined, bipedal, and possibly tool-using hominids in the late Miocene or early Pliocene, while Leakey (1967, 1968) has claimed that bones found in the Upper Miocene fossil beds of Fort Ternan, Kenya, show evidence of having been broken up or hammered by some kind of blunt instrument. It is true, as Bielicki points out, that

the possibility must be reckoned with that those hominids were not at all ancestral to the hominids known from the Pleistocene, but represented a result of a quite independently initiated, and for some reason "not completed" hominizing trend within one or more species of Tertiary catarrhines. Such a supposition would be in line with the . . . possibility that hominizing tendencies could have recurred several times in the history of other Primates, as well as with the well-known "dehumanization hypothesis" advanced by Kortlandt and Kooij (1963). [Bielicki 1969, p. 60]

However, the possibility remains that these earliest cultural ventures may have involved the use of bone and that this cultural tradition may have survived in some parts of the continent. In that event, the Makapansgat cultural manifestation may represent a late and perhaps final expression of such cultural activities, with a minimum incorporation of stone into the hardware of the material culture.

TEN

THE EARLY EXPRESSION OF STONE CULTURE

It has long been known that primitive stone tools were manufactured in Africa during australopithecine times. Opinion has been acutely divided, however, as to whether *Australopithecus* was their maker. In 1965, I gave a detailed review of the evidence as well as of the opinions for and against this hypothesis. It seemed to me then (1965d) and subsequently (1967a, 1968c, 1969b) that the balance of evidence was against *Australopithecus* having been the maker of the first systematic, cultural stone tools. My view agreed with that of Mason (1957, 1961, 1962) and of Robinson (1957, 1958, 1959, 1962a), as well as those of Inskeep (1959), von Koenigswald (1961, 1968), and others, that "*Australopithecus* is unlikely to have made the stone artefacts—it seems more likely that *Telanthropus* was responsible" (Robinson 1959, p. 585); and again, "It is not impossible, in view of the evidence accumulated by Dart, that *Australopithecus* had an 'osteodontokeratic' but not an established stone culture, but that *Telanthropus* did have the latter" (ibid., p. 585).

Some of the evidence was indirect or associational. Thus, speaking of the stone implements found in the Sterkfontein Middle Breccia, Mason stated:

It is unlikely that a complex technology would be practiced by australopithecines on one end of Africa and pithecanthropines on the other [the discoveries in Algeria and Morocco]. We have, therefore, good reason to suspect that pithecanthropines made the Sterkfontein [stone] artefacts and may have killed the australopithecine whose remains lie near the artefacts. Here we have the least speculative of all the varying interpretations that have been given to the Sterkfontein discoveries. We may not have to look to North Africa for a suitable hominid for, as J. T. Robinson has indicated, one lies at nearby Swartkrans in the form of *Telanthropus*. [Mason 1961, p. 14]

Since he has accepted the reassignation of *Telanthropus* as pithecanthropine, Mason states elsewhere that "we may now see [the australopithecines] as the unsuccessful competitors of progressive pithecanthropines who were making tools of Acheulean type" (Mason 1962, p. 124).

Robinson's evidence was likewise largely indirect and circumstantial.

His view was "that stone tools can only be attributed to australopithecines with any certainty if it is known that nothing more advanced was living at their time level" (Robinson 1962, p. 105). Spelled out more fully, this view is as follows:

If it can be proved that australopithecines occur in direct association with a stone industry over a significant period of time *when no evidence whatever exists of the presence at that level of anything more advanced than the australopithecines,* then there will be a sound case for regarding the australopithecines as tool-makers. In fact there is evidence throughout the entire australopithecine period either proving or suggesting the presence of a more advanced form of hominid. There are the large parietals in the "pre-Zinj" level of Olduvai, *"Telanthropus"* at Swartkrans associated directly with *Paranthropus,* and at Sangiran *"Pithecanthropus"* and *"Meganthropus"* occur in association. There is thus no period in the past in which australopithecines are known to occur in association with stone artefacts but about which all students are agreed that nothing more advanced than australopithecines occurs. [Robinson 1962a, p. 102]

I accept this argument in general (though not in all details; for instance, as applied to Indonesia, I do not consider that the case for an australopithecine there is yet proved). Accordingly, I followed up Robinson's statements with a detailed analysis of skeletal and cultural associations at a number of African sites (Tobias 1965d, 1965e). From some 15 sites, levels, or living floors analyzed, I was able to show that:

1. At every australopithecine locality with stone tools there is evidence of the coexistence of a more advanced hominid.

2. Wherever we find *Australopithecus* together with a more advanced hominid, there too we find stone tools.

3. Wherever early stone tools are found with hominid remains, the skeletal remains include a more advanced hominid, with or without *Australopithecus* as well.

4. Every early locality that has yielded a hominid more advanced than *Australopithecus* has stone tools in addition.

Although it is a dangerous procedure to speculate on the identity of the early stone tool maker in terms of negative evidence, it does seem to me that the evidence of these correlations from 15 localities may suggest a balance of probabilities. Unless we are to resort to a series of special pleas, the most reasonable hypothesis to explain these data would seem to be that *Australopithecus* was *not* the maker of the earliest cultural stone implements, but that more advanced hominids almost certainly were. The nature of such more advanced hominids is suggested by the recently described lowly hominine species, *Homo habilis,* from Olduvai Gorge (Leakey, Tobias, and Napier 1964), the habiline teeth found by Howell at Omo (1968), and gracile hominid remains from Lothagam and Koobi Fora near Lake Rudolph, as well as by the *Telanthropus* material from Swartkrans, which Simonetta (1957) and Robinson (1961) have re-allocated to *H. erectus,* but which I consider probably to belong to the same taxon as that to which *H. habilis* has been allocated. This applies, too, to the recently reconstructed hominine from Swartkrans (Clarke, Howell, and Brain 1970).

Tentatively, I have concluded from the direct evidence that *Australopithecus* was a tool user and that, at least in southern Africa, he made tools of bone, horn, and tooth, but only occasionally of stone.

The evidence from Olduvai is summarized with characteristic caution by Dr. Mary Leakey as follows:

. . . insofar as the hominid remains from Beds I and II are concerned, it must be stated that there is no direct evidence for linking any particular culture or cultural phase with any particular fossil skull. Both *H. habilis* and *Australopithecus* remains have been found on Oldowan and developed Oldowan living floors, and it is impossible to determine whether either or both represent the tenants of the camp sites or their victims. The position may be briefly summarized as follows:

Bed I and Lower Bed II:
No. 5 (*Zinjanthropus*), Nos. 6, 7, 8 (*H. habilis*), and No. 10 (?) found on Oldowan living sites.
No. 4 (*H. habilis*) and No. 16 (?) not associated with cultural material.
Middle and Upper Bed II:
No. 3 (australopithecine), No. 13 (? *H. habilis*), Nos. 14 and 15 (?) associated with the developed Oldowan.
No. 9 (*cf. H. erectus*) not associated with any culture.
No hominid remains are known either from Acheulian or Acheulian-developed Oldowan contact sites.

On the balance of evidence, none of which is conclusive, the repeated association of *H. habilis* and *Australopithecus* with the Oldowan and its derivative strongly suggests that one or the other must be responsible for that culture, with the scales tipped in favour of *H. habilis* on account of greater brain size and a degree of manual ability. It must be remembered, however, that the hand bones of the Olduvai australopithecines are not known. [M. D. Leakey 1967, 441–42]

Summation on Australopithecus and culture

When we combine the direct and indirect evidence, a general inference seems permissible. It is that *Australopithecus* was indeed characterized by greater cultural, no less than biological, hominization than the great apes. This cultural hominization expressed itself in the frequency and consistency of implemental patterns of behavior. In apes, tool-using and tool-making are infrequent, sporadic. The apes' way of life and survival do not depend upon such implemental means but rather on formidable natural defense mechanisms, and on a sheltered forest habitat.

Australopithecus, on the other hand, lived in a habitat providing little natural protection, and he had no natural weapons of offense, defense, and threat, like large canines. His implemental activities must have come to loom very largely in his pattern of adjustment. Indeed, it would not be too much to claim, on the basis of all the evidence that has been cited, that his very survival depended on implemental activities. This, I suggest, is the great step forward of *Australopithecus* over the apes. He learned to exploit a mental and manipulative capacity, a cultural potentiality, which even apes possess. And he exploited it so effectively that in time he and his offshoots became dependent on it for survival. Cultural capacity was the greatest evolutionary asset of *Australopithecus;* it was on this aspect of his form and function that selection operated with the greatest vigor. Already, in the economy of *Australopithecus,* there is evident that gradual transfer of emphasis from purely biological mechanisms to largely cultural modes of adaptation, which is the most striking feature of the subsequent evolution of man.

ELEVEN

 # THE TREND OF CULTURAL EVOLUTION

The facts and interpretations put forward above point to a long, sustained sequence of cultural development. We may recognize various stages in this sequence.

Pongids: sporadic, unsystematic implemental activity; limited horizon for problem-solving applications of implemental behavior; probably contributes only slightly, if at all, to survival.

Australopithecus: more versatile array of implemental activities; main media so far demonstrated bone, horn, and teeth—little desultory use of stone; incipiently systematic; of definite survival value; possibly a cul-de-sac of cultural evolution or, at least, difficult to show technological and typological continuity with the long lithic tradition.

Homo habilis: seemingly the first systematic, progressive, stone culture practitioners; implements of a set, regular pattern; numbers of patterns slowly increasing with diversifying tool-kit; degree of trimming on implements progressively increasing with advance from Oldowan to developed Oldowan cultures; continuity with ensuing (Acheulean) cultural phase easier to demonstrate; first indications of constructional activities; culture-dependence for survival is becoming a reality.

Homo erectus: where good cultural associations are present, manufacturers of advanced stone implements; Acheulean in Africa, a kind of developed Oldowan in Europe (Vértèsszöllös) and Asia (Choukoutien); sustained continuity of cultural development; consistency of patterns; diversification of tool types; first fire-making in places; possible dawn of ritual (Blanc 1961); survival value of culture is very high.

Homo sapiens: all significant trends of cultural hominization intensified: consistency, complexity, refinement, versatility, diversity within cultures, diversification between cultures with cultural adaptation; complex ritual life, with artistic manifestations; tolerance of wider range of human variants within the social group, leading to greater variability. Man is absolutely culture-dependent for survival.

Some features are difficult to place in such a taxonomic sequence. Where did hunting begin? Dart (1964 and many earlier references) is convinced that the transition from apehood to humanity was, as Darwin (1871) had suspected, predatory. According to this view, *Australopithecus* would have been a primitive hunter. Others have regarded *Homo erectus* as the first big-game hunter (cf. Krantz 1968). My own view is that *Australopithecus* and probably *Homo habilis* were primarily food-gatherers and scavengers with an element of facultative hunting, especially of young and weak or aged and infirm animals. As the armamentarium of *H. habilis* shows an improvement on that of *Australopithecus*, we may expect that predatory episodes would have become more common and that the taste for scavenged meat would have declined proportionately.

By the time *H. erectus* emerged, it seems that hunting had become a systematic, obligatory way of life, supplemented always of course by gathering. All the mental attributes necessary for sustained predaceous effort must have appeared.

Krantz has recently stressed the intimate relationship between brain development and hunting. Leaving aside desultory hunting activities, such as those that *Australopithecus* may have indulged in, Krantz concentrates his attention on what he calls *persistence hunting*, which he describes as "a uniquely human technique which is known to have been practiced recently by some primitive peoples." As examples, he cites the Tarahumara of Mexico, the Shoshonean Indians, and the Kalahari Bushmen. "In all of these cases of persistence hunting, the game is finally taken primarily because the hunter has been able to persist in the chase for as long as one or two days" (Krantz 1968, p. 450). Clearly, a most important requirement for persistence hunting, and one that is directly relevant to the development of the brain, is "the ability to keep the task constantly in mind for several days and to anticipate the results well into the future."

He cites Rensch and Altevogt (1955) as showing that memory is directly related to brain size, at least in their comparisons *between different species of animals*. In all cases, Rensch and his co-workers concluded, the species with the larger mean brain size proved to have the greater memory. Dobzhansky summarized their experiments in English and stated: "Rensch concludes that the memory retention is about proportional to the brain size in the animals experimented with by himself and his colleagues" (Dobzhansky 1962, p. 201). Krantz comments:

Judging from Rensch's observations, the increase of some 500 c.c. of endocranial volume in *Homo erectus* [as compared with *Australopithecus*] must certainly represent a tremendous increase in his memory. A brain at least ⅔ the size of modern man's brain should have permitted *H. erectus* to engage in persistence hunting in a manner approaching that observed in recent man.

The idea of persistence hunting permits the following hypothesis as to the selective forces that brought about the transformation from *Australopithecus* to *Homo:* small steps in the enlargement of the *Australopithecus* brain would have been of selective advantage mainly by increasing the time and distance that the possessor would be able to pursue his mobile food supply. Considering the young, injured, and aged as well as normal adults of all species of potential food available to our ancestors, there was a continuous gradation in pursuit times necessary to bring down game. At first, *Australopithecus* could run down only those animals most quickly exhausted, and must have been in keen competition with many other carnivores. As the reward in food for successful pursuit of game tended, on the average, to go to those individuals with the greater mental time spans, selective pressure would favour larger brains with better memories. [Krantz 1968, pp. 450–51]

A close look at this ingenious suggestion reveals the basic assumption Krantz has made, namely that because species with bigger brains (on the average) have better memories than other species with smaller brains, *within a species* individuals with bigger brains would be endowed with better memories than those individuals with smaller brains. I do not know of any experimental evidence to support this assumption at the intra-specific level. In fact, the problem seems analogous with the question of intelligence and brain size: within a species it has not proved possible to demonstrate valid genetic differences in intelligence or achievement between big-brained and small-brained variants (Tobias 1970). Unfortunately, if one questions Krantz's assumption, the edifice of his hypothesis likewise must be called into question.

All we can say is: (a) we need more information about the memory retention ability of big- and small-brained individuals *within a species,* and (b) memory may well be one, but only one, of a number of functions that have improved and increased with the development of greater internal structural complexity of the brain, which in turn has gone along with the increase in size of the brain. Selection for better memory may well be one of the selective pressures that favored larger brains during hominization. But there is no reason to believe it to be either the only one or even the main one.

Krantz himself suggested another mechanism of selection for increase of brain size—only this time not for the jump from *Australopithecus* to *H. erectus* but for that from *H. erectus* to *H. sapiens*. He was perplexed by the fact that cultural evolution moved so slowly during the "Lower Palaeolithic." How did it come about that a few simple stone implements such as hand axes and chopping tools persisted virtually unchanged for over a hundred thousand years? His hypothesis is based on the growth pattern of the hominid brain. This leads him to suggest that the small-brained Palaeolithic people *as adults* were as well endowed as their modern descendants, but that *as young children* they were incapable of the use of symbolic language. "This shortened the time available for acculturation and thus limited the culture content" (Krantz 1961, p. 85). Krantz accepts that "virtual humanity is reached with a normally developed brain in excess of the 750 c.c. threshold." Why then, he asks, do modern human brains average about 1400 c.c.? Why is there a further increase in average endocranial capacity of 65 per cent from *H. erectus* to *H. sapiens?* There does not seem to be any marked intellectual improvement, and we know that among modern people no clear correlation has been shown between brain size and intelligence. What advantage was gained by the additional, apparently superfluous increase?

He suggests an answer based on the growth pattern of the hominid brain. For the modern child, the value of 750 c.c. is reached at the end of the first year of life. According to Krantz:

> The child begins to use symbolic speech sometime during the following year, usually at about 18 months, though he may understand it several months earlier. It is here suggested that this minimum brain mass is just as necessary for the symbolizing ability in the individual ontogeny as it is in the phylogeny of man. While crossing the threshold does not guarantee speech if the nervous system is not adequately developed, this threshold sets a lower limit below which symbolizing is not possible. [Krantz 1961, p. 86]

Krantz then proceeds to draw a hypothetical curve of brain growth for *H. erectus,* setting the curve at a constant 61 per cent of the *H. sapiens* curve. The capacity of the Modjokerto child fits on this curve fairly well. The curve shows that the endocranial capacity of *H. erectus* did not pass the threshold of 750 c.c. until after the sixth year of life:

> Now, if the argument developed above is tenable, it is evident that the young *Pithecanthropus,* prior to the age of about six years, clearly did not possess the endocranial volume which appears to be a prerequisite for symbolization. Not until the age of six did the *Pithecanthropus* brain approach the volume and complexity of the brain of the modern one-year-old child. That this did in fact limit the mental abilities of these children seems to be an inescapable inference. [Ibid., p. 86]

Allowing for errors in the reconstruction of the *H. erectus* growth curve, the threshold crossing point could have been as low as four years or as high as eight years. According to Krantz, this point has previously eluded students of brain size, because juvenile capacities have been used thus far only as guides to the probable capacities of the adult skulls.

Increasing the size of the brain with the type of growth curve remaining constant results in a proportionate increase of the brain at all stages of life. Any increase thus moves the crossing of the threshold to a younger age. The advantage gained by this brain expansion is not to be found in the adult size, but in the gradual lowering of the age at which the children acquired the quantity of brain substance associated with symbolizing.

The enculturation of the individual is considered to be primarily, if not exclusively, based on the use of symbols. If the child lacks the ability to use and understand symbols until the age of six, his enculturation will be about five

141

years behind that of the normal modern child. When reproductive age was reached, the *Pithecanthropus* had no more than seven years of cultural experience, whereas when the modern man reaches reproductive maturity he has at least twelve years of cultural experience. Age estimates of known fossil men indicate a very low life expectancy as with modern hunters and gatherers. In this case, five years would be an appreciable portion of the lives of most individuals.

This shorter period of full cultural participation would limit the total quantity and complexity of cultural content that is likely to be transmitted in each generation. When the age of onset of symbolizing is lowered by increasing the child's brain size, the amount of cultural material that can be transmitted is increased. [Ibid., p. 86]

This interesting suggestion is put forward to explain the extraordinarily slow rate of change in the lower Palaeolithic. At the same time, it is suggested by Krantz that this may explain the large mass of superfluous brain tissue in modern man. The latter implication is predicated upon the assumption that *the pattern of brain growth would not have changed during evolution,* at least from *H. erectus* to *H. sapiens.* Yet, the pattern does differ appreciably between modern pongids and modern hominids (Zuckerman 1928; Keith 1931), the most notable difference being the steep initial postnatal rise in man, as compared with the apes. It is of course possible that there may have been a steady change in the curve of growth from the pongid pattern to the modern human curve during the several stages of hominization. From the nature of the material, however, the major changes are likely to have been at levels from pre-*Australopithecus* to *Australopithecus* to *H. habilis* to *H. erectus.* It is likely that, as Krantz assumes, the pattern of growth would have attained to something essentially similar to that of modern man by the time of *H. erectus.* In that event, his hypothesis would seem to be a valuable contribution to our thinking about brain sizes, ancient and modern.

Feedback

There has been much discussion in the literature as to the primacy of structural modifications or of behavioral changes during evolution. Thus, Washburn and Hamburg (1965), Washburn (1967), and Washburn and Shirek (1967) stress that behavior precedes structure in evolution. This in turn leads them to relegate a terminal role to the brain in human evolution. This view has been opposed by Holloway, who argues the converse, namely that the brain had a primary role in human evolution. It is obvious for him that "for any behavioral change to be evolutionary in significance, it must first rest upon an organic basis, underlain by a genetic change associated with the behavior; otherwise, evolution is impossible" (Holloway 1969a, p. 2).

Again, Holloway joins issue with Le Gros Clark when the latter states:

For it is not what animals *do* in their natural environment, but what they *can* do under changing and adverse conditions, that will ultimately determine how they will become adapted behaviourally, and finally physically, to new environments.

. . . progressive evolutionary development surely depends on deliberate efforts made by individual animals, and by the communities of which they are members, to overcome adverse and difficult problems with which they are faced in order to ensure the survival of the species. . . . If a species by such strivings can manage to survive for a sufficient length of time in surroundings for which it is not as yet fully adapted in its physical make-up, then the opportunity is provided for the gradual development by advantageous mutational variations of morphological changes that adapt the species more perfectly to its ecological environment. [Le Gros Clark 1967, pp. 121–22]

In his review of Le Gros Clark's *Man-Apes or Ape-Men?* Holloway comments, "This seems an unfortunate way to word the essential message: that plasticity of behavior was important in evolution. Left as it is, the statement is out of bounds with genetic and evolutionary theory" (Holloway 1968b, p. 422).

This kind of chicken-egg argument does not seem to be a particularly fruitful controversy. I find greater potential value in an approach that stresses the two-sidedness or reciprocity between genetico-structural bases and behavioral expressions. This relationship, modern thinking would indicate, is essentially a feedback one (Dobzhansky 1962, 1963; Bielicki 1964, 1965, 1969; Holloway 1967).

To quote Washburn and Howell:

Darwin and many workers after him stressed development of bipedal locomotion as a factor in differentiating man from ape. This process freed the hands, made possible the use and manufacture of tools, and led to reduction in the size of the teeth and the facial skeleton. The australopithecines in general represent such a stage in human evolution. [Washburn and Howell 1960, p. 35]

But they modify this view a page or two further on by commenting: "Perhaps, as Darwin suggested, tool use is both the cause and effect of hominid bipedalism, and the evolution of erect posture occurred simultaneously with the earliest use of tools" (ibid., p. 37).

These views remind us that there must have been a subtle reciprocal

143

feedback relationship between culture and its genetic bases, between physical and cultural evolution (Dobzhansky 1962, 1963; Bielicki 1964, 1965). "Did the genetic basis of culture appear before culture?" is a question we often hear asked (Tobias 1965d, p. 183). But Dobzhansky pointed out that this is a wrong way to ask the question; culture and its genetic basis developed, and are developing, together. Bielicki, following Washburn (1960), says:

It seems, for instance, that feedback between bipedalism and tool-using . . . was at work only in Pliocene protohominid apes, and faded out at the beginning of the Pleistocene, since in the Australopithecinae the process of acquiring bipedal gait had already been completed and further evolution of culture did not demand any further change in the mode of locomotion. [Bielicki 1964, p. 1]

On the other hand, the earlier sections of this volume have made clear that the brain-culture relationship was not confined to one special moment in time. Long-continuing increase in size and complexity of the brain was paralleled for probably a couple of millions of years by long-continuing elaboration and "complexification" (to use de Chardin's word) of the culture. The feedback relationship between the 2 sets of events is as indubitable as it was prolonged in time (Tobias 1969b).

Most recently, Bielicki (1969) has attempted a profound analysis of the causal interrelationships between the emergence and evolution of some of the anatomical, physiological and ecological peculiarities of hominids, and the origin and evolution of cultural behavior. To do this, he relies heavily on Maruyama's theory of deviation-amplifying cybernetic systems (1963). Bielicki lists the following traits, the evolution of which he regards as the essence of hominization:

Noncultural components

1. erect bipedal locomotion
2. various measures of brain size and complexity
3. noncyclic sexual receptivity of the female
4. retardation of ontogenetic development
5. predatory behavior (hunting)

Cultural components

6. implemental behavior (tool-using and tool-making)
7. symbolic communication
8. certain characteristics of social organization in which preagricultural humans most markedly diverged from subhuman catarrhines.

Bielicki develops the idea that, in the course of human evolution, there existed 2-directional causal links (feedbacks) between the noncultural and the cultural components. *These feedbacks were in each case positive,* that is, *deviation-reinforcing rather than homeostatic.* This is the crucial point stemming from Maruyama's theory.

For example, the interrelationship between the element "brain-size" A, and the element "complexity of implemental behavior," B, can be postulated to have been such that any progress in A must inevitably have led to some progress in B (because a shift of the frequency distribution of A "more to the right" would produce within the population a new extreme class of "supranormal" segregants who would, sooner or later, put to use their "extra capacities" and further enrich the existing technology). Contrariwise, any progress in B must have generated (by raising the proportion of "below-threshold" individuals in the population) selective pressures that, in turn, forced A to continue its development in the same direction as before. The 2 elements were bound to evolve together, in a parallel fashion, mutually stimulating one another.

Bielicki postulates the existence of such closed loops of positive feedbacks, sometimes in pairs, sometimes in triplets. Other combinations he considers are ontogenetic retardation–tool-making and erect bipedalism–tool-making–hunting. He thus attempts to conceive the whole process of hominization in terms of such deviation-amplifying or "morphogenetic" systems. Such systems exhibit certain properties that seem noteworthy to students of human evolution. For example, such a system is set in motion by an "initial kick," as stressed, too, by Holloway (1967), often small in extent and statistically, therefore, not at all improbable. Once initiated, the system would gradually and spontaneously build up deviations and diverge from the initial condition. Given enough time, a development can ensue that is disproportionately large as compared with the force of the initial push.

In other words,

. . . an insignificant, and therefore quite probable, deviation from a certain initial, static condition can, through the mutual amplification of deviations, finally result in a very considerable deviation which otherwise (i.e. without the existence of positive feedback circuits within the system) would have a very small probability of occurrence. [Bielicki 1969, p. 58]

Applying these ideas more specifically to human evolution, Bielicki suggests that the initial push may have been the emergence, in some species of Pliocene semiterrestrial pongids, of systematic tool-using and of rudimentary hunting. That is, the initial kick can be described as a slight deviation of the system from a condition of omnivorous food-gathering without tools or with only sporadic use of tools toward another condition, that of hunting and gathering with the systematic aid of unmodified tools. Maybe a single jump—or kick—to hunting is too great; the shift to scavenging, I should suggest, might be a more probable part of the first step. All the other features of hominization, as listed, could be interpreted as direct or indirect consequences of that initial "double-push." Thus, the direction of further evolution was determined at the very beginning of the whole process. The behavior of the whole system was characterized by a high degree of determination and predictability (Bielicki 1969).

A corollary, Bielicki points out, is that hominization is, in principle, a repeatable event. All that was needed was for the same initial kick to have occurred in several different species of higher catarrhines with similar structural and functional potentialities for tool-using and hunting (or scavenging). Thus, the early tool-using bipedal hominids postulated by Simons, Pilbeam, and Leakey to have existed in Mio-Pliocene times need not have been ancestral to the Pleistocene tool-users at all.

Another suggestion of Bielicki is that the process of hominization, once started, would soon have acquired a relatively high degree of independence of the stresses of the external environment, since it was not the external environment but cultural behavior that provided the main source of selective pressures on the population's genotype. One can therefore speculate, says Bielicki, that the whole process would not have stopped, and would have followed a fairly similar course, even in a completely static environment:

This seems to be a rather peculiar mode of evolution, different in certain respects from the standard situation in which the main driving force of long-term directional evolution of a species is a series of selective responses of the gene pool to the changing factors of the physical and biotic environment.

The above interpretation, however, has of course nothing to do with the concept of orthogenesis, since it does assume adaptation through natural selection as the principal agency responsible for the hominid evolutionary progression. [Bielicki 1969, p. 59]

Bielicki here seems to contradict himself. I shall return to this point below.

Another corollary, Bielicki believes, is that possibilities for extensive adaptive radiations with speciation within the hominid line can be presumed to have been very small.

Finally, he suggests that the hominization of the postcranial skeleton (especially the development of the structural basis for the bipedal gait) was an evolutionary response to the emergence of tool-using and hunting, these 3 trait-complexes being linked by a triplet of positive feedbacks.

Bielicki's conception represents an ingenious attempt to develop the notion of feedback and to provide a mechanism by which the very potent set of evolutionary pressures generated by the development of culture can play its part. It is clear that culture has come to play a dominant role in hominid evolution. Some ten years ago, in my presidential address to Section E of the South African Association for the Advancement of Science, I tried to develop this concept to explain rapid human evolution. Then, I suggested that when Cultural Selection and Natural Selection pull in the same direction, evolutionary change would be most rapid (Tobias 1961, pp. 33–36).

The notion was developed originally to explain steatopygia in the Bushmen—for this seemed to provide an excellent example of a selectively advantageous feature, the intensity of selection of which has been heightened by sexual or cultural pressures. The short size of the Bushmen was another phenotypic trait that seemed to be favored both for survival and by cultural preferences. The stronger the cultural pressures, the more drastic would be the cultural selection of certain qualities deemed desirable. If these qualities also assist the survival of the population, then both natural and cultural selection would operate in the same direction, and human evolution would proceed at a dramatically rapid tempo. The relevance of this example from micro-evolutionary change for the macro-evolutionary dimension of which Bielicki speaks is that it was suggested by me *not* that Cultural Selection ousted or supplanted Natural Selection, but that it *complemented* Natural Selection.*

Now, it seems to me that, excellent as is the hypothesis proposed by Bielicki, it errs by not allocating an adequate place to Natural Selection.

---

* Eiseley has drawn attention to the oft-overlooked Darwin-Wallace controversy on the mechanism of human evolution. While Darwin had adhered rigidly to Natural Selection as an adequate explanation of the rise of man and his brain, Wallace had realized that "some more rapid process of evolution than that envisaged in the Darwinian philosophy must have been at work in the production of man" (Eiseley 1956, p. 69). Seven years before *The Descent of Man,* Wallace had asserted that evolution in cultured man was largely mental, and that even racial differences were essentially survivals from the time when man was a still cultureless animal. However, he did not take the further step of postulating that this very culture had come to dominate selective processes in man. Instead, because he could envisage no other force to account for the rapid rise of the human brain, Wallace invoked a directive spiritual force that could not be accounted for in purely mechanistic terms.

Although he refers once to Natural Selection as *"the principal agency* responsible for the hominid evolutionary progression,"* yet a moment before he had been saying:

The process of hominization . . . soon acquired a relatively high degree of independence of the stresses exerted by the external environment, since it was not the external environment but cultural behaviour which provided *the main source* of selective pressures on the population's genotype. [Bielicki 1969, p. 59; italics mine]

There is an apparent contradiction between these statements; Doctor Bielicki cannot have his cake and eat it! Apart from this passing reference, the normal Natural Selective mechanism plays no part in the deviation-amplifying system elaborated in Bielicki's paper. The antinomy, I believe, can be resolved by bringing Natural Selection back into the picture. The positive feedback system could well have acquired a momentum of its own, whether or not the environmental stresses were changing; but if the positive feedback system in any way harmed the organism's survival chances, clearly Natural Selection would have acted subtly but definitely against the whole deviation-amplifying system—perhaps in favor of some homeostatic or alternative system that might have facilitated survival. In other words, I am suggesting that the whole operation of the deviation-reinforcing system was itself subject to Natural Selection. We are saying, in more cybernetic language, what I attempted to say in 1960, namely that all will be well as long as the culture-controlled mechanism and the natural selective mechanism are not at odds with each other.

A concrete example comes to mind: a positive feedback system between brain size (and what goes with it) and implemental behavior could have led to a substantial enhancement of brain size. If, however, such increased brain growth were spread more or less evenly over the entire period of immaturity, prenatal as well as postnatal (and not just postnatal, as Krantz, 1961, illustrated), a situation might have been reached where an increasing number of individuals would have had difficulty in giving birth to their large-headed babies. Increasing brain size, under these circumstances, would have been decidedly detrimental to survival. The deviation-amplifying system would have been powerless to overcome the hard fact that fewer babies were being born alive after protracted labors! In fact, this particular problem was overcome, not by an interruption of the positive feedback system but by a change in the pattern of brain growth. Instead of babies being born with 60 or 65 per cent of adult brain size, the percentage dropped to a much lower level: that is to say, the great bulk of ontogenetic expansion of the brain was delayed until after birth, when it ensued with dramatic suddenness. In other words, Natural Selection operated in favor of variants showing belated brain expansion—and in this way, the biological equipment was brought into line with the hungry demands of the positive feedback system.

POSTLUDE

This book has been more in the nature of an essay than a scientific treatise: for an essay sets out to explore ideas but does not necessarily prove anything! If one thing has been proven here, it is our need for much further information on many basic facts.

We have explored such facts as do exist on endocast size and have tried to add to the existing corpus of knowledge. We have made a few rudimentary attempts at computing population limits for various taxa of fossil hominids. We have shown that the greatest advance in mean cranial capacity apparently occurred between the Lower and Middle Pleistocene, with the emergence of *Homo erectus*.

On the other side of the coin, we have surveyed the evidence on cultural origins and early cultural growth. Here, too, we have seen that the most significant of the early cultural advances came with the rise and development of *Homo erectus*.

We were struck by the fact that of all the elements of hominization, 2 were alike in being long continued, sustained, and most marked: brain-size increase and cultural evolution. No other parameter for which adequate evidence is available equals these 2 in duration and continuity. We were constrained to probe below the surface, to seek the causal links between both ends of the chain leading from increased brain size to increased cultural complexity.

We considered the structural meaning of variations in brain size, both absolutely and in relation to body size. We spoke of neuron numbers and of internal reorganization of an enlarging brain, and examined the interrelations of the various parameters. We realized that the area between the hard factual extremes (endocasts and implements) was a shadowy, twilight zone of controlled speculation. We saw that a few venturesome souls are trying to throw light on this gloomy zone and thereby to rationalize the causal steps between brain size and tools. While pausing to doff our caps at them, we concluded that both termini of our causal chain were worthy objects of study in their own right, as long as we observe due restraint in the functional and behavioral interpretations we make from them.

So we moved on, to retrace the evolutionary story on the cultural side: we explored the limitations of the world of the apes, the awakening dawn of *Australopithecus,* the settling in of *Homo habilis,* the maturation of *Homo erectus,* and the flowering and prospering of *Homo sapiens.*

We tried to dissect the various trends of cultural hominization, as we had earlier done of brain-size increases. And we invoked the aid of cybernetics to explore some of the 2-way relationships between cultural and non-cultural features.

When accepting the invitation to deliver this James Arthur Lecture, I intended to learn something about brain evolution. All the way along, I had the guiding words of Claude Bernard echoing in my ear: "It is what we *think* we know that prevents us from learning."

Every so often, I had to steel myself, being mindful of Wilfred Trotter's words, written long before the days of Professor Christiaan Barnard: "The mind likes a strange idea as little as the body likes a strange protein and resists it with a similar energy" (Trotter 1941, p. 186).

Finally, at the end of it all, I found myself retreating to the potted opiate of James Thurber, whom I shall allow to have the last word:

The brain of our species is, as we know, made up largely of potassium, phosphorus, propaganda, and politics, with the result that how not to understand what should be clearer is becoming easier and easier for all of us. Sanity, soundness, and sincerity, of which gleams and stains can still be found in the human brain under powerful microscopes, flourish only in a culture of clarification, which is now becoming harder and harder to detect with the naked eye. [Thurber 1961, pp. 112–13]

REFERENCES

Anderson, J. H. (1910). "The proportionate contents of the skull." *Jl. R. anthrop. Inst.,* **xi.**

Appel, F. W., and E. M. Appel (1942). "Intracranial variation in the weight of the human brain." *Hum. Biol.,* **14** (1–2), 48–68, 235–50.

Ariens Kappers, C. U., and H. Bouman (1939). "Comparison of the endocranial casts of the *Pithecanthropus erectus* skull found by Dubois and von Koenigswald's *Pithecanthropus* skull." *Proc. K. ned. Akad. Wet.,* **42**, 30–40.

Ashton, E. H. (1950). "The endocranial capacities of the *Australopithecinae.*" *Proc. zool. Soc., Lond.,* **120**, Part IV, 715–21.

Ashton, E. H., and T. F. Spence (1958). "Age changes in the cranial capacity and foramen magnum of hominoids." *Proc. zool. Soc., Lond.,* **130**, 169–81.

Bailey, P., and G. von Bonin (1951). *The Isocortex of Man.* Urbana: University of Illinois Press.

Bauchot, R., and H. Stephan (1967). "Encéphales et moulages endocraniens de quelques Insectivores et Primates actuels." *Problèmes Actuels de Paléontologie (Évolution des Vertébrés)* (163), 575–86. Éditions du Centre National de la Recherche Scientifique.

Beatty, H. (1951). "A note on the behaviour of the chimpanzee." *J. Mammal.,* **32**, 118.

Bielicki, T. (1964). "Evolution of the intensity of feedbacks between physical and cultural evolution from man's emergence to present times." UNESCO Expert Meeting on the Biological Aspects of Race, Moscow, 12–18 August 1964 (manuscript), pp. 1–3.

—— (1966). "On *Homo habilis.*" *Curr. Anthrop.,* **7** (5), 576–78.

—— (1969). "Deviation-amplifying cybernetic systems and hominid evolution." *Mater. i Pr. Anthrop.* (77), 57–60.

Bielicki, T., and A. Wanke (1965). "Wczesnoplejstoceńskie Hominidy Z Olduvai I Zagadnienie 'Bocznych Odgalezień' W Ewolucji Cztowieka." *Kosmos A, Warsz.,* **XIV** (1), 31–43.

Blanc, A. C. (1961). "Some evidence for the ideologies of early man." In S. L. Washburn (ed.), *Social Life of Early Man.* Chicago: Aldine Publishing Company, pp. 119–36.

Blinkov, S. M., and I. I. Glezer (1968). *The Human Brain in Figures and Tables.* New York, Basic Books and Plenum Press.

Bolk, L. (1904). "Beziehungen zwischen Hirnvolum und Schädelcapazität, nebst Bermerkungen über das Hirngewicht der Holländer." *Petrus Camper ned. Bijdr. Anat.,* **ii**, 511–36.

———— (1925). "On the existence of a dolichocephalic race of gorilla." *Proc. K. ned. Akad. Wet.*, **28** (2), 204–13.

Bolwig, N. (1961). "An intelligent tool-using baboon." *S. Afr. J. Sci.*, **57** (6), 147–52.

Bonin, G. von (1934). "On the size of man's brain as indicated by skull capacity." *J. comp. Neurol.*, **59** (1), 1–28.

———— (1948). "The frontal lobe of Primates: cytoarchitectural studies." *Res. Publs. Ass. Res. nerv. ment. Dis.*, **27**, 67–83.

———— (1963). *The Evolution of the Human Brain*. Chicago: University of Chicago Press.

Boule, M., and H. V. Vallois (1957). *Fossil Men*. New York: The Dryden Press.

Boyd, R. (1861). "Tables of the weights of the human body and internal organs in the sane and insane of both sexes at various ages arranged from 2614 postmortem examinations." *Phil. Tr. R. Soc.*, **151**, 241–62.

Brain, C. K. (1967). "The Transvaal Museum's fossil project at Swartkrans." *S. Afr. J. Sci.*, **63** (9), 378–84.

———— (1968). "Who killed the Swartkrans ape-men?" *S. Afr. Mus. Assoc. Bull.*, **9** (4), 127–39.

———— (1970). "New finds at the Swartkrans Australopithecine site." *Nature, Lond.*, **225** (5238), 1112–18.

Brandes, K. (1927). "Liquorverhältnisse an der Leiche und Hirnschwelling." *Frankf. Z. Path.*, **35**, 274–301.

Breitinger, E. (1936). "Zur messung der Schädelkapazität mit Senfkörnern." *Anthrop. Anz.*, **13**, 140–48.

Broom, R. and J. T. Robinson (1948). "Size of the brain in the ape-man, *Plesianthropus*." *Nature, Lond.*, **161** (4090), 438.

———— (1952). "Swartkrans ape-man, *Paranthropus crassidens*." *Transv. Mus. Mem.* (6).

Broom, R., J. T. Robinson, and G. W. H. Schepers (1950). "Sterkfontein ape-man, *Plesianthropus*." *Transv. Mus. Mem.* (4).

Broom, R., and G. W. H. Schepers (1946). "The South African fossil ape-men, the Australopithecinae." *Transv. Mus. Mem.* (2).

Campbell, B. G. (1962). "The systematics of man." *Nature, Lond.*, **194** (4825), 225–32.

———— (1963). "Quantitative taxonomy and human evolution." In S. L. Washburn (ed.), *Classification and Human Evolution*. Chicago: Viking Fund Publications in Anthropology, pp. 50–74.

Clark, W. E. Le Gros (1947). "Observations on the anatomy of the fossil *Australopithecinae*." *J. Anat.*, **81** (3), 300–33.

———— (1964). *The Fossil Evidence for Human Evolution*. Second edition. Chicago: University of Chicago Press.

———— (1965). "There is a transcendence from Science to Science." Second Raymond Dart Lecture. Johannesburg: Institute for the Study of Man in Africa and Witwatersrand University Press, pp. 1–18.

—— (1967). *Man-apes or Ape-men? The Study of Discoveries in Africa.* New York: Holt, Rinehart & Winston.

Clark, W. E. Le Gros, D. M. Cooper, and S. Zuckerman (1936). "The endocranial cast of the chimpanzee." *Jl. R. anthrop. Inst.* **66** (II), 249–68.

Clarke, R. J., F. C. Howell, and C. K. Brain (1970). "More evidence of an advanced hominid at Swartkrans." *Nature, Lond.,* **225** (5239), pp. 1219–22.

Cobb, S. (1965). "Brain size." *Archs. Neurol. Chicago.* **12**, 555–61.

Connolly, C. J. (1950). *External Morphology of the Primate Brain.* Springfield, Ill.: Thomas.

Cooke, H. B. S. (1963). "Pleistocene mammal faunas of Africa, with particular reference to Southern Africa." In F. C. Howell and F. Bourlière (eds.), *African Ecology and Human Evolution.* New York: Wenner-Gren Foundation. (Viking Fund Publications in Anthropology, no. 36.)

Coon, C. S. (1963). *The Origin of Races.* London: Jonathan Cape.

Dart, R. A. (1925). "*Australopithecus africanus:* the man-ape of South Africa." *Nature, Lond.,* **115** (2884), 195–99.

—— (1926). "Taungs and its significance." *Nat. Hist., N. Y.,* **26**, 315–27.

—— (1929). "A note on the Taungs skull." *S. Afr. J. Sci.,* **26**, 648–58.

—— (1956a). "The relationship of brain size and brain pattern to human status." *S. Afr. J. med. Sci.,* **21** (1–2), 23–45.

—— (1956b). "Cultural status of the South African man-apes." *Rep. Smithson. Instn., 1955,* 317–38.

—— (1957). "The osteodontokeratic culture of *Australopithecus prometheus.*" *Transv. Mus. Mem.* (10).

—— (1962). "The Makapansgat pink breccia australopithecine skull." *Am. J. phys. Anthrop.,* **20** (2), 119–26.

—— (1964). "The ecology of the South African man-apes." In D. H. S. Davis (ed.), *Ecological Studies in Southern Africa. Monographiae biol.* Vol. XIV, The Hague: W. Junk, pp. 49–66.

Darwin, C. (1871). *The Descent of Man.* 2 vols. London: Murray.

Dobzhansky, T. (1962). *Mankind Evolving: the Evolution of the Human Species.* New Haven: Yale University Press.

—— (1963). "Cultural direction of human evolution—a summation." *Hum. Biol.,* **35** (3), 311–16.

Donaldson, H. H. (1895). *The Growth of the Brain.* London: Walter Scott, Ltd.

Donisthorpe, J. (1958). "A pilot study of the mountain gorilla (*Gorilla gorilla beringei*) in South West Uganda, February to September, 1957." *S. Afr. J. Sci.,* **54** (8), 195–217.

[Dubois, E. (1895)]. Dr. Dubois' "Missing Link." Report on his address to a meeting of the Royal Dublin Society, 20 November 1895. *Nature, Lond.,* **53**, 115–16.

Dubois, E. (1898). "Remarks upon the brain-cast of *Pithecanthropus erectus.*" *Proc. IVth Int. Congr. Zool., Cambridge, 1898,* 85–86.

—— (1918a). "On the relation between the quantities of the brain, the neurone and its parts, and the size of the body." *Proc. K. ned. Akad. Wet.,* 20 (9–10), 1328–37.

—— (1918b). "Comparison of the brain-weight in function of the body-weight, between the two sexes." *Proc. K. ned. Akad. Wet.,* 21 (6–7), 850–69.

—— (1919). "The significance of the size of the neurone and its parts." *Proc. K. ned. Akad. Wet.,* 21 (5), 711.

—— (1920). "The quantitative relations of the nervous system determined by the mechanism of the neurones." *Proc. K. ned. Akad. Wet.,* 22 (7–8), 665–80.

—— (1921). "On the significance of the large cranial capacity of *Homo Neandertalensis.*" *Proc. K. ned. Akad. Wet.,* 23 (8), 1271–88.

—— (1922). "On the cranial form of *Homo Neandertalensis* and of *Pithecanthropus erectus,* determined by mechanical factors." *Proc. K. ned. Akad. Wet.,* 24 (6–7), 313–32.

—— (1924). "On the brain quantity of specialised genera of mammals." *Proc. K. ned. Akad. Wet.,* 27 (5–6), 430–37.

—— (1933). "The shape and the size of the brian in *Sinanthropus* and in *Pithecanthropus.*" *Proc. K. ned. Akad. Wet.,* 36 (4), 415–23.

—— (1934). "Phylogenetic cerebral growth." *Int. Congr. anthrop. ethnol. Sci.,* 71–74.

Edinger, T. (1948). "Evolution of the horse brain." *Mem. geol. Soc. Am.,* 25, 1–177.

Eiseley, L. (1956). "Fossil man and human evolution." In W. L. Thomas, Jr. (ed.), *Current Anthropology.* Chicago: University of Chicago Press, pp. 61–78.

—— (1958). *The Immense Journey.* New York: Random House, Inc.

Gaul, G. (1933). "Über die Wachstumveränderungen am Gehirn-Schädel des Orang-utan. *Z. Morph. Anthrop.* 31, 362–94.

Goodall, J. (1963a). "Feeding behaviour of wild chimpanzees." *Symp. zool. Soc., London* (10), 39–47.

—— (1963b). "My life among wild chimpanzees." *Natn. geogr. Mag.,* 124 (2), 272–308.

—— (1964). "Tool-using and aimed throwing in a community of free-living chimpanzees." *Nature, Lond.,* 201 (4926), 1264–66.

Greenfield, J. G., and E. A. Carmichael (1925). *The cerebrospinal fluid in clinical diagnosis.* London: Macmillan.

Gyldenstolpe, N. (1928). "Zoological results of the Swedish expedition to Central Africa, 1921." Vertebrata 5, *Ark. Zool.,* 20A, 1–76.

Hagedoorn, A. (1924). "Schedelcapaciteit van Anthropomorphen." *Ned. Tijdschr. Geneesk.,* 68 (Part 1, No. 11), 1240–42.

—— (1926). "Schädelkapazität der Anthropomorphen." *Anat. Anz.,* 60 (18), 417–27.

Harris, H. A. (1926). "Endocranial form of gorilla skulls with special reference to the existence of dolichocephaly as a normal feature of certain primates." *Am. J. phys. Anthrop.,* 9 (2), 157–72.

Hayes, C. (1952). *The ape in our house.* London: Victor Gollancz Ltd.

Holloway, R. L. (1965). "Cranial capacity of the hominid from Olduvai Bed I." *Nature, Lond.,* **208** (5006), 205–206.

—— (1966a). "Cranial capacity of the Olduvai Bed I hominine." *Nature, Lond.,* **210** (5041), 1108–09.

—— (1966b). "Cranial capacity, neural re-organization, and hominid evolution: a search for more suitable parameters." *Am. Anthrop.,* **68,** 103–21.

—— (1967). "The evolution of the human brain: some notes towards a synthesis between neural structure and the evolution of complex behaviour." *Gen. Syst.,* **12,** 3–19.

—— (1968a). "The evolution of the Primate brain: some aspects of quantitative relations." *Brain Res.,* **7,** 121–72.

—— (1968b). "Review of *Man-Apes or Ape-Men? The Story of Discoveries in Africa,* by Sir Wilfrid E. Le Gros Clark." *Hum. Biol.,* **40** (3), 421–23.

—— (1969a). "The role of the brain in human mosaic evolution." Paper presented to *VIII Int. Congr. anthrop. ethnol. Sciences,* Tokyo and Kyoto, 3–10 Sept., 1968.

—— (1969b). "Some questions on parameters of neural evolution in Primates." *Ann. N. Y. Acad. Sci.,* **167** (1), 332–40.

—— (1970a). "Neural parameters, hunting, and the evolution of the human brain." In C. R. Noback and W. Montagna (eds.), *Advances in Primatology; Vol. 1: The Primate Brain.* New York: Appleton-Century-Crofts, pp. 299–310.

—— (1970b). "Australopithecine endocast (Taung specimen, 1924): a new volume determination." *Science, N. Y.,* **168,** 966–68.

Howell, F. C. (1965). "Comment on Olduvai hominids." *Curr. Anthrop.,* **6** (4), 399–401.

—— (1968). "Omo Research Expedition." *Nature, Lond.,* **219** (5154), 567–72.

Hunt, J. (1863). "On the Negro's Place in Nature." *Anthrop. Soc. of London,* 17th November 1863. London: Trubner and Co., pp. 1–64.

Inskeep, R. R. (1959). "Central and West Africa: Prehistory." *Encyclopaedia Britannica.* London: William Benton, pp. 328–30.

Jacob, T. (1964). "A new hominid skull cap from Pleistocene Sangiran." *Anthropologica,* N.S. **VI** (1), 97–104.

—— (1966). "The sixth skull cap of *Pithecanthropus erectus.*" *Am. J. phys. Anthrop.,* **25** (3), 243–60.

Jerison, H. J. (1963). "Interpreting the evolution of the brain." *Hum. Biol.,* **35** (3), 263–91.

Keith, A. (1895). "The growth of brain in man and monkeys." *J. Anat. Physiol., Lond.,* **29,** 282–303.

—— (1925). "The fossil anthropoid ape from Taungs." *Nature, Lond.,* **115** (2885), 234–35.

—— (1931). *New Discoveries Relating to the Antiquity of Man.* London: Williams and Norgate.

Khroustov, G. F. (1968). Formation and highest frontier of the implemental activity of anthropoids. *VII Int. Congr. anthrop. ethnol. Sci.,* Moscow, 3–10 August 1964. Vol. 3, 503–509.

Kirchner, G. (1895). "Der Schädel des *Hylobates concolor,* sein Variationskreis und Zahnbau." Inaugural Dissertation, Univ. Erlangen, pp. 1–55.

Klüver, H. (1937). "Re-examination of implement-using behaviour in a Cebus monkey after an interval of three years." *Acta psychol.,* **2,** 347–97.

Koenigswald, G. H. R. von (1961). "*Australopithecus* und das Problem der Geröllkulturen." *Dt. Ges. Anthrop.,* 7. Tagung Tübingen, April 1961, 139–52.

―――― (1967). "Neue Dokumente zur Menschlichen Stammegeschichte." *Eclog. geol. Helv.,* **60,** 641–55.

―――― (1968a). "Probleme der ältesten menschlichen Kulturen." Aus *Handgebrauch und Verstandigung bei Affen und Fruhmenschen.* Bern und Stuttgart: Verlag Hans Huber. 149–73.

―――― (1968b). "The numbering of the *Pithecanthropus* skulls." *Proc. K. ned. Akad. Wet.,* **271** (B), 408.

Köhler, W. (1924). *The Mentality of Apes.* New York: Vintage Books, 1959 (English edition).

Kohts, N. (1935). "Infant ape and human child (instincts, emotions, play, habits)." *Trudȳ zoopsikhol. Lab. gos. darvin. Muz.*

Kortlandt, A. (1962). "Chimpanzees in the wild." *Scient. Am.,* **206,** 128–38.

Kortlandt, A., and M. Kooij (1963). "Protohominid behaviour in Primates." *Symp. zool. Soc. Lond.* (10), 61–87.

Krantz, G. S. (1961). "Pithecanthropine brain size and its cultural consequences." *Man,* **11** (103), 85–87.

―――― (1968). "Brain size and hunting ability in earliest man." *Curr. Anthrop.,* **9** (5), 450–51.

Krompecher, St., and J. Lipak (1966). "A simple method for determining cerebralization: brain weight and intelligence." *J. comp. Neur.,* **127** (1), 113–20.

Kummer, B. (1961). "Beitrag zur quantitativen Bestimmung der Entwicklungshöhe des Säugetiergehirnes." *Psychiatria Neurol.,* **142,** 352–75.

Lashley, K. S. (1949). "Persistent problems in the evolution of mind." *Q. Rev. Biol.,* **24,** 28–42.

Latimer, H. B. (1950). "The weights of the brain and of its parts and the weight and length of the spinal cord in the adult male guinea pig." *J. comp. Neurol.,* **93** (1), 37–51.

Leakey, L. S. B. (1959). "A new fossil skull from Olduvai." *Nature, Lond.,* **184** (4685), 491–93.

―――― (1960). "Recent discoveries at Olduvai Gorge." *Nature, Lond.,* **188** (4755), 1050–52.

―――― (1961). "New finds at Olduvai Gorge." *Nature, Lond.,* **189** (4765), 649–50.

―――― (1966). "*Homo habilis, Homo erectus* and the australopithecines." *Nature, Lond.,* **209** (5030), 1279–81.

—— (1967). "Development of aggression as a factor in early human and pre-human evolution." In C. D. Clemente and D. B. Lindsley (eds.), *Aggression and Defence: Neural Mechanism and Social Patterns; Vol. 5: Brain Function*. Berkeley and Los Angeles: University of California Press, pp. 1–33.

—— (1968). "Bone smashing by late Miocene Hominidae." *Nature, Lond.,* **218** (5141), 528–30.

Leakey, L. S. B., and M. D. Leakey (1964). "Recent discoveries of fossil hominids in Tanganyika: at Olduvai and near Lake Natron." *Nature, Lond.,* **202** (4927), 5–7.

Leakey, L. S. B., P. V. Tobias, and J. R. Napier (1964). "A new species of the genus *Homo* from Olduvai Gorge." *Nature, Lond.,* **202** (4927), 7–9.

Leakey, M. D. (1967). "Preliminary survey of the cultural material from Beds I and II, Olduvai Gorge, Tanzania." In W. W. Bishop and J. D. Clark (eds.), *Background to Evolution in Africa*. Chicago: University of Chicago Press, pp. 417–46.

Lindley, D. V., and J. C. P. Miller (1953). *Cambridge Elementary Statistical Tables*. Cambridge: Cambridge University Press.

Marchand, F. (1902). "Über das Hirngewicht des Menchsen." *Abh. sächs. Akad. Wiss.,* **27**, 391–482.

Maruyama, M. (1963). "The second cybernetics: deviation-amplifying mutual-causal processes." *Am. Scient.,* **51**, 164–79.

Mason, R. J. (1957). "Occurrence of stone artefacts with *Australopithecus* at Sterkfontein, Part II." *Nature, Lond.,* **180** (4585), 521–24.

—— (1961). "The earliest tool-makers in South Africa." *S. Afr. J. Sci.,* **57** (1), 13–16.

—— (1962). "Australopithecines and artefacts at Sterkfontein, Part II. The Sterkfontein stone artefacts and their maker." *S. Afr. archaeol. Bull.,* **17** (66), 109–25.

Matiegka, H. (1902). "Über das Hirngewicht, die Schädelkapazität und die Kopf-form, sowie deren Beziehungen sur psychischen Thätigkeit des Menschen." *Sber. K. böhm. Ges. Wiss.* (20), 1–75.

Merfield, F. G. (1956). *Gorillas were my neighbours*. London: Longmans, Green and Co.

Mettler, F. A. (1955). "Culture and the structural evolution of the neural system." *James Arthur Lecture on the Evolution of the Human Brain*. New York: American Museum of Natural History.

Napier, J. R. (1960). "Studies of the hands of living Primates." *Proc. zool. Soc. London,* **134** (4), 647–57.

Nissl, F. (1898). "Nervenzellen und graue Substanz." *Munch. med. Wschr.,* **45**, 988.

Olivier, G. (1971). "Estimation of the standard deviation for hominid cranial capacity." (Unpublished manuscript, personal communication)

Oppenheim, S. (1911–1912). "Zur Typologie des Primatencraniums." *Z. Morph. Anthrop.,* **14**, 1–204.

Osborn, R. (1963). "Observations on the behaviour of the mountain gorilla." *Symp. zool. Soc., Lond.* (10), 29–37.

Osman Hill, W. C. (1960). "Cebidae," Parts A and B. *Primates.* Vols. 4 and 5. Edinburgh: Edinburgh University Press.

Owen, R. (1866). *Comparative Anatomy and Physiology of Vertebrates.* London: Longmans, Green, and Co.

Pakkenberg, H., and J. Voigt (1964). "Brain weight of the Danes." *Acta anat.,* **56** (4), 297–307.

Pearl, R. (1905). "Biometrical studies in man. I. Variation and correlation in brain weight." *Biometrika,* **4**, 13–104.

Pfister, H. (1903). "Die Kapazität des Schädels beim Säugling und älteren Kinde." *Mschr. Psychiat. Neurol.,* **13**, 577–89.

Pilbeam, D. R. (1969). "Early Hominidae and cranial capacity." *Nature, Lond.,* **224**, 386.

Pilbeam, D. R., and E. L. Simons (1965). "Some problems of hominid classification." *Am. Scient.,* **53** (2), 237–59.

Pineau, H. (1965). "La croissance et ses lois." Thèse doct. Sci., Paris.

Radinsky, L. (1967). "Relative brain size: a new measure." *Science, N. Y.,* **155** (3764), 836–38.

—— (1968). "A new approach to mammalian cranial analysis, illustrated by examples of prosimian Primates." *J. Morph.,* **124** (2), 167–80.

Randall, F. E. (1943–1944). "The skeletal and dental development and variability of the gorilla." *Hum. Biol.,* **15** (3–4), 236–54, 307–37; **16** (1), 23–76.

Rensch, B., and R. Altevogt (1955). "Das Ausmäss visueller lernfähigkeit eines Indischen Elefanten." *Z. Tierpsychol.,* **12** (1).

Robinson, J. T. (1952). "The australopithecines and their evolutionary significance." *Proc. Linn. Soc. Lond.,* **3**, 196–200.

—— (1954). "The genera and species of the *Australopithecinae." Am. J. phys. Anthrop.,* **12** (2), 181–200.

—— (1956). "The dentition of the *Australopithecinae." Transv. Mus. Mem.* (9).

—— (1957). "Occurrence of stone artefacts with *Australopithecus* at Sterkfontein." *Nature, Lond.,* **180** (4585), 521–24.

—— (1958). "The Sterkfontein tool-maker." *Leech, Johannesb.,* **28** (4–5), 94–100.

—— (1959). "A bone implement from Sterkfontein." *Nature, Lond.,* **184** (4686), 583–85.

—— (1960). "The affinities of the new Olduvai australopithecine." *Nature, Lond.,* **186** (4723), 456–58.

—— (1961). "The australopithecines and their bearing on the origin of man and of stone tool-making." *S. Afr. J. Sci.,* **57** (1), 3–13.

—— (1962a). "Australopithecines and artefacts at Sterkfontein. Part I: Sterkfontein stratigraphy and the significance of the Extension Site." *S. Afr. archaeol. Bull.,* **17** (66), 87–107.

—— (1962b). "The origin and adaptive radiation of the australopithecines." In G. Kurth (ed.), *Evolution und Hominisation*. Stuttgart: Gustav Fischer.

—— (1965). "*Homo 'habilis'* and the Australopithecines." *Nature, Lond.*, **205**, 121–24.

—— (1966). "The distinctiveness of *Homo habilis*." *Nature, Lond.*, **209**, 957–60.

—— (1968). Addendum to "The origin and adaptive radiation of the Australopithecines." In G. Kurth (ed.), *Evolution und Hominisation*. Second edition. Stuttgart: Gustav Fischer.

Rudolph, O. (1914). "Untersuchungen über Hirngewicht, Hirnvolumen und Schädelkapazität." *Beitr. path. Anat.*, **58**, 48–87.

Sacchetti, A. (1942). Über die relative Variabilität des anthropometrischen Merkmale. *Z. Rassenk.*, **13**, 63–68.

Sartono, S. (1964). "On a new find of another pithecanthropine skull: an announcement." *Bull. geol. Surv. Indonesia*, **1** (1), 2–5.

—— (1967). "An additional skull cap of a *Pithecanthropus*." *Zinruigaku zassi. J. anthrop. Soc. Japan*, **75** (754).

—— (1968). "Early man in Java: *Pithecanthropus* skull VII, a male specimen of *Pithecanthropus erectus* (I)." *Proc. K. ned. Akad. Wet.*, **71B** (5), 396–422.

—— (1970). *The discovery of a hominid skull at Sangiran, Central Java*. Special Publication No. 3 of Geological Survey of Indonesia, 1–11.

—— (1971). "Some cranial measurements of *Pithecanthropus VIII*." Pending.

Schaller, G. B. (1963). *The Mountain Gorilla: Ecology and Behavior*. Chicago: University of Chicago Press.

Schepers, G. W. H. (1946). *See* Broom and Schepers (1946).

—— (1950). *See* Broom, Robinson, and Schepers (1950).

Schreider, E. (1966). "Brain weight correlation calculated from original results of Paul Broca." *Am. J. phys. Anthrop.*, **25** (2), 153–58.

Schultz, A. H. (1933). "Observations on the growth, classification and evolutionary specializations of gibbons and siamangs." *Hum. Biol.*, **5** (2–3), 212–55, 385–428.

—— (1944). "Age changes and variability in gibbons. A morphological study on a population sample of a man-like ape." *Am. J. phys. Anthrop.*, **2** (1), 1–129.

—— (1962). "Die Schädelkapazität männlicher Gorillas und ihr Höchstwert." *Anthrop. Anz.*, **25** (2–3), 197–203.

—— (1965). "The cranial capacity and the orbital volume of hominoids according to age and sex." *Homenaje a Juan Comas en su 65 anniversario*. Vol. II. Editorial Libros de México.

Schwalbe, G. (1902). "Über die Beziehungen zwischen Innenform und Aussenform des Schädels." *Dt. Arch. klin. Med.*, **73**, 359–408.

Selenka, E. (1896). "Die Rassen und der Zahnwechsel des Orang-utan." *Sber. dt. Akad. Wiss.* (quoted by Zuckerman, 1928).

—— (1898). *Studien über Entwickelungsgeschichte der Tiere*. Heft 6: Menschenaffen (Anthropomorphae). Studien über Entwickelung und Schädelbau. I.

Rassen, Schädel und Bezahnung des Orangutan. Wiesbaden: C. W. Kreidel, pp. 1–91.

—— (1899). *Studien über Entwickelungsgeschichte der Tiere.* Heft 7: Menschenaffen (Anthropomorphae). Studien über Entwickelung und Schädelbau. II. Schädel des Gorilla und Schimpanse. Wiesbaden: C. W. Kreidel, pp. 95–160.

Shariff, G. A. (1953). "Cell counts in the primate cerebral cortex." *J. comp. Neurol.,* **98** (3), 381–400.

Sholl, D. A. (1956). *The Organization of the Cerebral Cortex.* London: Methuen and Co.

Simon, E. (1965). "Endocranium, Endokranialausguss und Gehirn beim einhöckerigen Kamel (*Camelus dromedarius*)." *Acta anat.,* **60** (1), 122–51.

Simonetta, A. (1957). "Catalogo e sinonimia annotata degli ominoidi fossili ed attuali (1758–1955)." *Atti Soc. tosc. Sci. nat. Pisa,* **64** (B), 53–112.

Simpson, G. G., A. Roe, and R. C. Lewontin (1960). *Quantitative Zoology.* Revised edition. New York: Harcourt Brace Jovanovich.

Siwe, S. A. (1931). "Das Nervensystem." In *Handbuch der Anatomie des Kindes.* Vol. 2, pp. 590–728.

Sollas, W. J. (1926). "A sagittal section of the skull of *Australopithecus africanus.*" *Q. Jl. geol. Soc. Lond.,* **82,** 1–11.

Spann, W., and H. O. Dustmann (1965). "Das menschliche Hirngewicht und seine Abhângigkeit von Lebensalter, Körperlange, Todesursache und Beruf." *Dt. Z. ges. gericht. Med.,* **56,** 299–317.

Stephan, H. (1969). "Quantitative investigations on visual structures in primate brains." *Proc. 2nd int. Congr. Primat., Atlanta, Ga. 1968, 3,* 34–42. Basel, Karger/New York.

Stillman, C. K. (1911). "Edema of the pia-arachnoid." *Archs. intern. Med.,* **viii** (2), 193–239.

Suradi, T. (1965). "Laporan singkat tentung penemuan tengkorak *Pithecanthropus* VII." Unpublished report of the Geological Survey of Indonesia (quoted by Sartono 1968).

—— (1969). *"Pithecanthropus VIII* (?), sebuah laporan singkat tentang penemuannja" [*Pithecanthropus VIII* (?), a short report of its discovery]. Unpublished report of the Geological Survey of Indonesia (quoted by Sartono 1970).

Tabulae Biologicae (1941). Vol. 20: *Growth of Man.*

Thurber, J. (1961). *Lanterns and Lances.* London: Hamish Hamilton.

Tobias, P. V. (1961). "New evidence and new views on the evolution of man in Africa." *S. Afr. J. Sci.,* **57** (2), 25–38.

—— (1963). "Cranial capacity of *Zinjanthropus* and other Australopithecines." *Nature, Lond.,* **197** (4869), 743–46.

—— (1964). "The Olduvai Bed I hominine with special reference to its cranial capacity." *Nature, Lond.,* **202** (4927), 3–4.

—— (1965a). "Reply to R. L. Holloway: Cranial capacity of the hominine from Olduvai Bed I." *Nature, Lond.,* **208** (5006), 206.

—— (1965b). "New discoveries in Tanganyika: their bearing on hominid evolution." *Curr. Anthrop.,* **6** (4), 391–99.

—— (1965c). "*Homo habilis:* last missing link in hominine phylogeny?" In S. Genoves (ed.), *Festschrift on 65th birthday of Professor Juan Comas.* Vol. II. Editorial Libro de Mexico.

—— (1965d). "*Australopithecus, Homo habilis,* tool-using and tool-making." *S. Afr. archaeol. Bull.,* **20** (80), 167–92.

—— (1965e). "The early *Australopithecus* and *Homo* from Tanzania." *Anthropologie, Prague,* **3** (3), 43–48.

—— (1966a). "The distinctiveness of *Homo habilis.*" *Nature, Lond.,* **209** (5027), 953–57.

—— (1966b). "On *Homo habilis:* Reply to T. Bielicki." *Curr. Anthrop.,* **7** (5), 579–80.

—— (1967a). *Olduvai Gorge;* Vol. II: *The Cranium and Maxillary Dentition of Australopithecus (Zinjanthropus) boisei.* Cambridge: Cambridge University Press.

—— (1967b). "General questions arising from some lower and middle Pleistocene hominids of the Olduvai Gorge, Tanzania." *S. Afr. J. Sci.,* **63** (2), 41–48.

—— (1968a). "The taxonomy and phylogeny of the Australopithecines." In B. Chiarelli (ed.), *Taxonomy and Phylogeny of Old World Primates, with References to the Origin of Man.* Supplement to 1967 Volume of *Rivista di Antropologia.* Turin: Rosenburg and Sellier, pp. 277–315.

—— (1968b). "Cranial capacity in anthropoid apes, *Australopithecus* and *Homo habilis,* with comments on skewed samples." *S. Afr. J. Sci.,* **64** (2), 81–91.

—— (1968c). "Cultural hominization among the earlier African Pleistocene hominids." *Proc. prehist. Soc.,* N. S. **33,** 367–76.

—— (1969a). "Bigeneric nomina: a proposal for modification of the Rules of Nomenclature." *Am. J. phys. Anthrop.,* **31** (1), 103–106.

—— (1969b). *Man's Past and Future.* Fifth Raymond Dart Lecture. Johannesburg: Institute for the Study of Man in Africa and Witwatersrand University Press.

—— (1970). "Brain size, grey matter and race—fact or fiction?" *Am. J. phys. Anthrop.,* **32** (1), 3–26.

—— (1971). "Early man in Southern and Eastern Africa." Paper presented to Burg Wartenstein Symposium No. 48 on "Functional and Evolutionary Biology of Primates: Methods of Study and Recent Advances," July 18–26, 1970, pp. 1–39.

Tobias, P. V., and G. H. R. von Koenigswald (1964). "Comparison between the Olduvai hominines and those of Java and some implications for hominid phylogeny." *Nature, Lond.,* **204** (4958), 515–18.

Todd, T. W. (1923). "Dura volume in the male White skull." *Anat. Rec.,* **26** (4), 263–73.

Tower, D. B. (1954). "Structural and functional organisation of mammalian cerebral cortex. The correlation of neurone density with brain size." *J. comp. Neurol.,* **101** (1), 19–53.

Tower, D. B., and K. A. C. Elliott (1952). "Activity of the acetylcholine system in the cerebral cortex of various unanaesthetised mammals." *Am. J. Physiol.,* **168** (3), 747–59.

Trotter, W. R. (1941). *The Collected Papers of Wilfred Trotter F. R. S.* Oxford: Oxford University Press.

Vallois, H. V. (1954). "La capacité crânienne chez les Primates supérieurs et le 'Rubicon cérébral.'" *C. r. Acad. Sci. Paris,* **238,** 1249–51.

Vevers, G. M., and J. S. Weiner (1963). "Use of a tool by a captive capuchin monkey (*Cebus appela*)." *Symp. zool. Soc. Lond.* (10), 115–17.

Vlček, E. (1969). *Neandertaler der Tschechoslowakei.* Praha: Academia.

Washburn, S. L. (1960). "Tools and human evolution." *Scient. Am.,* **203,** 63–75.

———— (1967). "Perspectives and prospects." *Am. J. phys. Anthrop.,* **27** (3), 367–75.

Washburn, S. L., and D. A. Hamburg (1965). "The study of primate behavior." In I. de Vore (ed.), *Primate Behavior.* New York: Holt, Rinehart & Winston.

Washburn, S. L., and F. C. Howell (1960). "Human evolution and culture." In S. Tax (ed.), *Evolution after Darwin; Vol. II: The Evolution of Man.* Chicago: University of Chicago Press.

Washburn, S. L., and J. Shirek (1967). "Human Evolution. II." In J. Hirsch (ed.), *Behavior-Genetic Analysis.* New York: McGraw-Hill.

Weidenreich, F. (1936). "Observations on the form and proportions of the endocranial casts of *Sinanthropus pekinensis,* other hominids and the great apes: a comparative study of brain size." *Palaeont. sin. D.* **7** (4), 1–50.

———— (1941). "The brain and its role in the phylogenetic transformation of the human skull." *Trans. Am. phil. Soc.,* **31** (Part V), 321–442.

———— (1943). "The skull of *Sinanthropus pekinensis.*" *Palaeont. sin.* **127,** 1–486.

———— (1946). *Apes Giants and Man.* Chicago: University of Chicago Press.

Weiner, J. S. (1963). *See* Vevers and Weiner (1963).

Weinert, H. (1928). *"Pithecanthropus erectus." Z. Anat. EntwGesch.* **87,** 429–547.

Woo, J. K. (1965). "Preliminary report on a skull of *Sinanthropus lantianensis* of Lantian, Shensi." *Scientia Sin.,* **14,** 1032–35.

Yerkes, R. M. (1948). *Chimpanzees.* Fourth edition. New Haven: Yale University Press.

Zuckerman, S. (1928). "Age-changes in the chimpanzee, with special reference to growth of brain, eruption of teeth, and estimation of age; with a note on the Taungs ape." *Proc. zool. Soc. Lond.,* Part 1, 1–42.

INDEX

Acheulian tools, 134, 136, 138

Age estimates of fossil man, 142

Altevogt, R., 139, 160

Anderson, J. H., 10, 153

Appel, F. W. and E. M., 10, 153

Ariens Kappers, C. U., 87, 153

Art, dawn of, 138

Arthur, James, Lecture, v, vii

Ashton, E. H., 15, 20, 26, 33, 36–43, 46, 69–71, 153

Asselar, 100

Atlanthropus mauritanicus, see H. erectus mauritanicus

Australopithecus, 4, 96, 109, 112, 124–39; *africanus,* 2, 3, 19–21, 59, 65, 67–68, 73, 80–81, 96–98, 110–11; *boisei,* 4, 24–26, 65–66, 73, 110–11, 136; *robustus,* 21–24, 111, 135; ecology of, 124–25, 133, 137; functional aspects of, 125–27; morphology of, 125–26, 137; cultural activities of, 127–39

Baboon behavior, 117, 120; crania, fractured, 130–31

Bailey, P., 31, 114, 153

Bauchot, R., vii, 153

Beatty, H., 119, 153

Behavior, 113–14; evolution of, 113, 142 ff.; cultural, of non-hominid Primates, 116–24; learned, 125; genetic changes and, 142–43

Bernard, C., 152

Bielicki, T., 58, 72, 116, 133, 143–48, 153

Bischoff, T. L. W., 36, 38

Blanc, A. C., 138, 153

Blinkov, S. M., 11, 153

Bolk, L., 10, 39, 43, 153–54

Bolwig, N., 117, 154

Bone tools, *see under* Tools

Bonin, G. von, viii, 31, 100, 102, 104, 113–14, 153–54

Boskop, 100

Boule, M., 87, 91, 154

Bouman, H., 87, 153

Boyd, R., 14, 154

Brain, C. K., 23–24, 132, 136, 154–55

Brain: areas of, vii; convolutions of, vii; fissures of, vii; lobes of, vii; sulci of, vii–viii, 114; degree of fissuration of, viii, 114; reorganization of, 113–15; functional patterns, 114–15

Brain size: vii, 2–3, 144; evolutionary increase in, viii, 96–103, 114–15, 139–40, 142–43; age changes, 10–11, 68–71, 139; in illness, 10; growth, 11, 14–15, 26, 68–71, 140–42, 148; and selective pressures, 99–103, 115, 139–40, 146; evolutionary decrease in, 100–3; and culture, 101, 125, 136, 145, 148; and ability, 102, 105, 140–41; structure and, 103 ff., 115, 125–26; and behavior, 104–5, 113, 115–16, 125, 140–41; and body size, 106–8, 110; intraspecific variation of, 107, 140; of Caucasoids, 108; of Negroes, 108; as a morphological feature, 113, 116; and hunting, 139–40; and memory, 139–40; "superfluous," 142

Brandes, K., 9, 11, 154

Breitinger, E., 8, 154

Broca, P., 108

Broken Hill, 93, 100